Third Edition

SHARED GOVERNANCE

A Practical Approach to Transforming Interprofessional Healthcare

Diana Swihart
PhD, DMin, MSN, APN CS, RN-BC

Robert G. Hess, Jr.
RN, PhD, FAAN
Founder of the Forum for Shared Governance

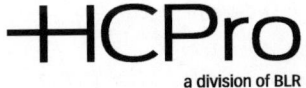

Shared Governance, Third Edition is published by HCPro, a division of BLR

Copyright © 2014 HCPro, a division of BLR

The Index of Professional Nursing Governance (IPNG) and Index of Professional Governance (IPG) are included by permission, and are copyright © 2014 Robert G. Hess, Jr.

All rights reserved. Printed in the United States of America.   5   4   3   2   1

Download the additional materials of this book at *www.hcpro.com/downloads/12207*

ISBN: 978-1-55645-114-0

No part of this publication may be reproduced, in any form or by any means, without prior written consent of HCPro or the Copyright Clearance Center (978-750-8400). Please notify us immediately if you have received an unauthorized copy.

HCPro provides information resources for the healthcare industry.

HCPro is not affiliated in any way with The Joint Commission, which owns the JCAHO and Joint Commission trademarks. MAGNET™, MAGNET RECOGNITION PROGRAM®, and ANCC MAGNET RECOGNITION® are trademarks of the American Nurses Credentialing Center (ANCC). The products and services of HCPro are neither sponsored nor endorsed by the ANCC. The acronym "MRP" is not a trademark of HCPro or its parent company.

Diana Swihart, PhD, DMin, MSN, APN CS, RN-BC, Author

Robert G. Hess, Jr., RN, PhD, FAAN, Author

Claudette Moore, Acquisitions Editor

Rebecca Hendren, Product Manager

Erin Callahan, Senior Director, Product

Elizabeth Petersen, Vice President

Matt Sharpe, Production Supervisor

Vincent Skyers, Design Manager

Vicki McMahan, Sr. Graphic Designer

Jason Gregory, Layout/Graphic Design

Mike King, Cover Designer

Advice given is general. Readers should consult professional counsel for specific legal, ethical, or clinical questions.

Arrangements can be made for quantity discounts. For more information, contact:

HCPro

75 Sylvan Street, Suite A-101

Danvers, MA 01923

Telephone: 800-650-6787 or 781-639-1872

Fax: 800-639-8511

Email: *customerservice@hcpro.com*

Visit HCPro online at: *www.hcpro.com* and *www.hcmarketplace.com*

Contents

Dedication ix

Acknowledgments xi

About the Authors xiii

Preface xv

Foreword xix

Chapter 1: Introduction 1

Chapter 2: Design a Structure to Support Shared Governance 15

Chapter 3: Build a Structure to Support Shared Governance 27

Chapter 4: Building the Practice and Unit Councils 51

Chapter 5: Implementing Shared Governance at the Organization Level 73

Chapter 6: Measuring Shared Governance 79

Chapter 7: Interprofessional Shared Governance in Healthcare 87

Chapter 8: Case Studies 105

Chapter 9: Relationships for Excellence 129

Chapter 10: Tips for Success 149

Chapter 11: The Forum for Shared Governance 157

Chapter 12: Conclusions and Recommendations 161

Appendix A: Shared Governance Measurement Tools: IPNG and IPG 165

Appendix B: Expanded Bibliography 175

To access the tools and sample documents included in this book
and its appendixes, visit the link below.

www.hcpro.com/downloads/12207

List of Figures

Figure 1.1: Four characteristics of the principles of shared governance 5

Figure 1.2: Self-governance vs. shared governance 8

Figure 1.3: Benefits and challenges of shared governance 11

Figure 1.4: Moving from a hierarchy to relational partnership 12

Figure 2.1: Systems descriptions 16

Figure 2.2: Sample health system model 17

Figure 2.3: Interdisciplinary shared governance model 17

Figure 2.4: Interdisciplinary shared governance process model 18

Figure 2.5: Characteristics of accountability and responsibility 19

Figure 2.6: The congressional model of shared governance 21

Figure 2.7: The councilor model of shared governance 23

Figure 2.8: The administrative model of shared governance 24

Figure 2.9: Unit or practice microsystem 25

Figure 3.1: Strategic changes related to implementing shared governance 29

Figure 3.2: ARCTIC assessment tool 31

Figure 3.3: Shared governance steering group functions and tasks 37

Figure 5.1: From management to leadership 77

Figure 7.1: Cincinnati Children's similar but separate governance structures 92

Figure 7.2: Cincinnati Children's interprofessional shared governance model 96

Figure 7.3: Cincinnati Children's interprofessional practice model 97

Figure 7.4: Cincinnati Children's nursing cluster coordinating structure 99

Figure 7.5: Cincinnati Children's shared leadership model 102

Figure 7.6: Cincinnati Children's facilitator responsibilities 105

Figure 8.1: Beaumont Nurse Professional Practice Model 112

Figure 8.2: Beaumont shared governance model 113

Figure 8.3: Beaumont council membership application 119

Figure 8.4: Scorecard for Beaumont council membership application 121

Figure 8.5: Beaumont shared governance organizational overview 122

Figure 8.6: KHCC professional practice model 124

Figure 8.7: KHCC unit-based council model 125

Figure 8.8: KHCC shared governance structure 126

List of Online Appendixes

Appendix 1	Index of Professional Governance (IPG)
Appendix 2	Index of Professional Nursing Governance (IPNG)
Appendix 3	Comparing Features Shared Governance
Appendix 4	Council Shared Decision-Making Tool
Appendix 5	Competency Decision Worksheet
Appendix 6	Competencies in Shared Governance
Appendix 7	Quality Commitment Agreement
Appendix 8	Clinical Quality Champion Orientation
Appendix 9	Bylaws & Guidelines
Appendix 10	Council Role Descriptions
Appendix 11	Central Council Bylaws
Appendix 12	Unit Practice Council Charter
Appendix 13	Shared Governance Council Consult Form
Appendix 14	Council Communications Policy
Appendix 15	Communication Flow Chart
Appendix 16	Council Attendance Report

Appendix 17	Council Minutes 2	
Appendix 18	Council Agenda Minutes Template	
Appendix 19	Unit Practice Council Minutes 1	
Appendix 20	Council Sign-in Form	
Appendix 21	Performance Improvement	
Appendix 22	Peer Evaluation Tool	
Appendix 23	AAR	
Appendix 24	Guide to Journal Clubs	
Appendix 25	Council SWOT Strategic Planning	
Appendix 26	Strategic Planning Tool	
Appendix 27	Council Strategic Planning	
Appendix 28	Unit Practice Council Worksheet	
Appendix 29	Unit Practice Ground Rules	
Appendix 30	Council Discussion Planner	
Appendix 31	Council Quarterly Report	
Appendix 32	Council Team Building	
Appendix 33	Activities in Progress Form	
Appendix 34	Conflict Resolution Worksheet	
Appendix 35	HCP Shared Governance Bill of Rights	
Appendix 36	Influencing Style Interview	
Appendix 37	Shared Governance 2013 Articles Research	
Appendix 38	Comprehensive Bibliography	

Dedication

To those who have the passion and willingness to give back to others; those who understand the importance of giving. Judie Bopp best expressed the specialty of preceptoring and its impact on those who give and receive within the context of such relationships: "The capacity to watch over and guard the well-being of others is an important gift, and one that is learned with great difficulty. For it is one thing to see the situation others are in, but it is quite another to care enough about them to want to help, and yet another to know what to do."

—Diana Swihart

To the staff, managers, and executives in all healthcare professions who passionately believe that the best possible professional, organizational, and patient outcomes can only be achieved by empowering everyone to share in decision-making about patient care. To staff for trying something new and risky, to managers for trading traditional roles for unknown new ones, and to executives for supporting staff and managers and showing the way.

—Robert G. Hess, Jr.

Acknowledgments

Every work, regardless of scope and size, is completed only with the help and inspiration of others. My sincere thanks go to my beloved husband, Dr. Stan, for his support and encouragement, his unwavering belief in me.

I would also like to acknowledge those many nurses and other healthcare providers, patients and community partners, speakers and teachers, and colleagues and friends who have contributed their ideas and thoughts through countless classes, seminars, lectures, and discussions over the years. I write from their influence and want to recognize their contributions as well. Though their names are too numerous to list, many others can be found in this work and in the extended bibliography. To each and every one of you, thank you.

Finally, I would like to thank two innovative and courageous leaders who have most transformed my own thinking about shared governance: Dr. Robert Hess, a friend and colleague who taught me to measure shared governance and how to see more clearly the potential for nurses to truly lead change and advance healthcare on every level; and Dr. Tim Porter-O'Grady, whose work first drew me to the study of shared governance and continues to inspire my own work. After studying more than 180 articles, videos, and books, my ideas and writing most strongly reflect Dr. Porter-O'Grady's influence. For this reason, I am particularly pleased both of these extraordinary nurses have participated in writing what I hope to be another valuable addition to your own journey in helping reshape and transform professional practice in healthcare for this and the next generation.

—*Diana Swihart, PhD, DMin, MSN, APN CS, RN-BC*

I would first like to acknowledge the voice of reason in my life: my wife and partner of 40 years, Evamaria Eskin, MD. One night while going to bed, when I was perseverating about my dissertation ideas, Evi turned to me and said, "Why don't you propose something you know something about?" And that led me to defining and measuring shared governance.

I am eternally grateful to Tim Porter-O'Grady, DM, EdD, ScD (h), FAAN, one of my sponsors into the American Academy of Nursing, a mentor, and a resonant soundboard for my incessant questions. It was Tim who first challenged me to solidify my conceptual thinking to quantify shared governance and share the data.

I also want to acknowledge my partner in shared governance, Diana Swihart, PhD, DMin, MSN, APN CS, RN-BC. We make quite a lively team, with my irreverence and her torrent of proper energy. As I sail around in a conceptual stratosphere, I can see Diana beckoning me to return to the weeds where the real work is done. And I thank her for that. She has taught me a lot.

Finally, I have been privileged to work with some of the most fascinating and empowering healthcare professionals on earth, both during my hospital career (read: before *Nursing Spectrum* magazine) and my more than 20 years with the Gannett Healthcare Group, my present day job. To every nurse and allied healthcare professional who has schooled me about real-life experiences with implementing shared governance, thank you for keeping me grounded.

I know this looks like a round robin to Diana's acknowledgements, but that's just the way it is.

—*Robert Hess, RN, PhD, FAAN*

About the Authors

Diana Swihart, PhD, DMin, MSN, APN CS, RN-BC

Dr. Diana Swihart, the CEO for the American Academy for Preceptor Advancement, enjoys many roles in her professional career, practicing in widely diverse clinical and nonclinical settings. An author, speaker, researcher, educator, and consultant, she has published and spoken nationally and internationally on a number of topics related to preceptors, shared governance, competency assessment, professional development, servant leadership, Magnet Recognition Program®, research, and evidence-based practice. In 2008, her publication *Nurse Preceptor Program Builder: Tools for a Successful Preceptor Program* (2nd ed.) was selected as a foundational resource for the national VHA RN Residency Program.

Dr. Swihart has served as an ANCC Magnet Recognition Program® accreditation appraiser, as the treasurer for the National Nursing Staff Development Organization, and as adjunct faculty at South University and Trinity Theological Seminary and College of the Bible distance learning program.

Robert G. Hess, Jr., RN, PhD, FAAN

Robert G. Hess, Jr., RN, PhD, FAAN, is an educator, editor, author, consultant, and the founder of the Forum for Shared Governance. He currently serves as executive vice president of global programming for Gannett Education. An award-winning author, he has written more than 100 articles for numerous journals and books. He is the former vice chair of ANCC's Commission on Accreditation.

In 2008, Dr. Hess was inducted as a fellow into the American Academy of Nursing for his work in shared governance.

Preface

Shared governance structures, with all of their intrinsic complexities, responsibilities, and accountabilities, must be carefully designed and implemented to be sustained. This book takes some of the guesswork out of the various structures and processes behind shared governance and provides strategies, case examples, and best practices to make the daily operations of shared governance meaningful and successful. It is designed to provide a broad base on which to build planning and implementation of a successful shared governance infrastructure. To do that, you need guides, tips, and tools.

The purpose of the third edition of *Shared Governance* is to provide leaders, educators, and healthcare providers with many of the essential tools and ideas for practical approaches for designing—or redesigning—an effective and efficient interprofessional and multidisciplinary shared governance process model. They will facilitate your ability to embrace the evolving changes needed to mature your shared governance infrastructure towards sustainment. In this book you will find a compilation of information and tools to help you develop your own models and processes.

Quality, continual improvement, and excellence are embedded in healthcare practices across disciplines and services as the demand for value, safety, effectiveness, and efficiency grow and expand, directed at achieving outcomes that measure and increase the value of processes, i.e., shared governance. Therefore, this book also explores the relationship between shared governance and the American Nurses Credentialing Center (ANCC) Magnet Recognition Program® (MRP) and the International Organization of Standards (ISO) outlining the MRP, as well as ISO expectations for shared governance practices.

You will also find guides for identifying models and tools for designing and building a structure to support shared governance. Additional tools help you create your structures from the unit or practice level upwards and mature your processes across disciplines and service lines.

You can explore ways to engage internal and external stakeholders, assess your processes and outcomes, and evaluate your infrastructure within six domains of measurement. This book helps you as you grow and develop your knowledge, skills, and abilities through research, evidence-based practice, and shared decisional processes. These tools can support your work as you participate in a partnership with your leadership, educators, interprofessional colleagues, and multidisciplinary team members to ensure safe, competent practice within your organization.

Let's take a closer look and see what's here.

Organization

This edition of *Shared Governance* is organized into 12 chapters with strategic and tactical processes for implementing your own organizational management system. This work explores the evolving processes and decisions folded into shared governance. The book contains a plethora of field-tested tools, measurement instruments, and strategies to help guide steering groups, for designing and redesigning unit and practice councils, and to support governing (or central) councils. Each chapter begins with an encouraging quote and concludes with a brief summary of content.

- Chapter 1 explains the concept behind shared governance in today's complex work and healthcare environments. It looks at four primary principles of shared governance (partnership, equity, accountability, and ownership) and compares several models.
- Chapter 2 identifies some of the characteristics of shared governance structures and structural process models. Basic guidelines for forming governance bodies provide further insight into designing a structure to support shared governance within the organization and across service lines.
- Chapter 3 explores four components for building a structure to support shared governance in diverse work settings. Part one speaks to implementing shared governance. Part two discusses leading strategic change. Part three considers shared governance systems' perspective and format in designing the structures. Part four guides you through the process for formalizing the shared governance structure with bylaws and articles. This chapter also offers a brief look at redesigning shared governance after a breakdown in implementation has occurred.

- Chapter 4 focuses on building the practice and unit councils at points of service. Strategies and tools encourage providers to create a critical forum for participating in shared decisional processes and outcomes specific to their needs and activities.

- Chapter 5 describes the process for implementing shared governance at organizational levels. Building strong interprofessional and multidisciplinary relationships with key stakeholders, e.g., leadership, union representatives, community members, providers, staff, and patients, are critical to integrating shared governance into the organization.

- Chapter 6 identifies research projects specific to the principles and newest instruments used to measure shared governance, i.e., the Index of Professional Governance 2.0 (IPG) and the Index of Professional Nursing Governance 2.0 (IPNG).

- Chapter 7 relates one healthcare organization's strategic priorities, successes, rewards, and challenges of implementing an integrated interprofessional shared governance system across disciplines and services.

- Chapter 8 offers snapshots of shared governance in case studies contributed by organizations in two U.S. and global communities.

- Chapter 9 explores quality, safety, and value in quality management systems and service excellence through shared governance. Experts in the implementation of ISO 9001:2008 quality management and in the ANCC's MRP provide insight into how these systems complement and are more fully realized through shared governance.

- Chapter 10 offers tips for success, lessons learned, and best practices shared by healthcare leaders, direct-care providers, team leaders, and other organizations and communities of practice where shared governance thrives.

- Chapter 11 features an international clearinghouse for research and resources with examples of recent published and unpublished research on shared governance.

- Chapter 12 considers conclusions and recommendations for going forward with shared governance. Lived shared governance is a dynamic, fluid, and ever-growing process that can transform healthcare. You have the book, the tools, and a foundation built by many of your colleagues, peers, and thought leaders. All that remains is to determine how you will answer the question, "Where do we go from here?"

The information presented in *Shared Governance, Third Edition*, reflects the research and opinions of the authors, contributors, and advisors. Because of ongoing research and improvements in interprofessional and multidisciplinary team structures, information technology, and education, this information, these tools, and their applications are constantly shifting, changing, and evolving in healthcare, leadership, and other services and disciplines.

Because this book explores opportunities for folding shared governance into increasingly complex adaptive and uncertain work environments, we have provided you with definitions, a variety of models and tools, and multiple approaches to building stronger infrastructures within your own organization. It is the authors' sincere hope you will add this work to your library and consider how you, too, might contribute to this growing body of knowledge, research, and expertise through your own practice and organizational development.

—Diana Swihart and Robert G. Hess, Jr.

Foreword

The concept of shared governance continues to be a centerpiece of developing the collaborative environment for patient care. It continues to address the need to engage and empower people, which is the centerpiece of shared governance. Shared governance has been associated with good management for some 60 years. It seems to many that such concepts are new and innovative simply because so few leaders actually implement these concepts into the exercise of their own management. The prevailing model for management has historically been one that represents parent-child relationships, because it is the predominant model of leadership that most people can identify in the absence of real leadership education.

In nursing, much of management represents a parental and maternal influence that extends into the staff management interaction at every level of nursing practice. From the orientation program to policy, procedure, protocols, and practices, the nurse is constantly reminded of how much his or her life is scripted and controlled by external parameters and directives. It is no wonder that, given enough time, most nurses lose interest in controlling their own practice and influencing the practice lives of others. Ultimately, a nurse's locus of control becomes so narrow that he or she ceases to do anything but the most functional and routine activities and quickly becomes addicted to the predictable and ritualistic activities of nursing.

It is a challenge to get nurses out of their rut and fully engage them in their practice lives. Even when it is clearly in the best interest of the nurse to become more fully involved, the vagaries of work, the demands of patient care, and any other excuse becomes the barrier to fully engaging with those things that are necessary to advance and change practice. The leaders, for their part, have created such a vertical orientation and relationship that staff ultimately feel as though anything significant, important, or valuable can only be done by managers or by management mandate. They feel that any effort on the part of the staff infringes on their time and therefore is not legitimate. In this age of reform and interdisciplinary integration around an evidence-driven patient care model, the engaged and mature partnership role of the nurse is the essential centerpiece.

Shared governance reflects a completely different mental model for relationship and for leadership within and between disciplines. It recognizes that nursing as a profession coordinates, integrates, and facilitates the interface between the disciplines and around the patient. In fact, shared governance is predominantly about building a particular infrastructure or framework for building an effective interprofessional interaction between nursing and its care partners. It reorients the decision-making construct to require a broader distribution of decisions across the professions and allocates decisions based on accountability and role contributions to the collective work of patient care. This reconfiguration of the health system is intended to define staff-based decisions, accountability, roles, and ownership of all clinical staff in those activities that directly affect the care of the patient.

Success with shared governance requires a powerful reorientation of the organization. It requires leadership to understand that a significant retooling of leadership capacity and skill is required to successfully implement shared governance and sustain it as a way of life in the professional organization. Implementing shared governance means retraining managers, engaging staff, reallocating accountability, and building a truly staff-driven model of decision and action. Because behavior cannot be changed or sustained without a supporting infrastructure, it means redesigning and structuring the organization to eliminate rewards for passive behavior and enumerating and inculcating rewards for engagement within the very fabric of the organization.

Staff-driven decision-making is a strong indicator of excellence. It is no surprise that the American Nurses Credentialing Center Magnet Recognition Program® bases its major themes in a way that reflects the values and system of shared governance and staff-based accountability. Also, the work is not easy, and it cannot be done overnight. It means building an entire new culture that clearly and unambiguously reflects the characteristics of a truly collaborative, professional organization. From the highest levels of organizational leadership to the patient relationship, there must be strong evidence of practice driving the organization's work. In all professions, power is grounded in practice. Excellence in practice can only be obtained and sustained if the practitioners hold and exercise the power that only practice can drive in achieving excellence and satisfaction. Without it, the power to influence, change, challenge, and "push the walls" toward innovation and creativity is simply vacated, and others end up playing that role, whether their doing so is legitimate or not.

Sharon Finnigan and I wrote the first definitive book on shared governance in 1985. Although we and others have continued to add to that body of knowledge over the years, no substantial foundational text on implementing the basics of an effective shared governance system has been forthcoming since that time, until this current work (written first in 2006, expanded in 2011 and 2014). Here, the author has clearly enumerated the foundations of shared governance and the practical elements necessary to construct a shared governance structure (including the interdisciplinary requisites) and to make it successful. This is perhaps one of the clearest explications of the principles, design, and processes associated with a viable and successful shared governance model that exists in the literature today.

If the reader carefully works through this text and thoughtfully reasons and applies the principles set out herein, he or she can advance the opportunity to create a successful approach to broad-based shared governance. Each stage of development, every design element, each component of the decision process, and each evaluation of effectiveness outlined here provides the tools necessary to make implementation successful. Although the work will be focused and sometimes difficult, the rewards have proven to be substantial to those who have been willing to risk the effort and initiate the dynamic of creating a truly professional patient-centered organization. There is no greater indicator of a viable and sustainable potential for nurses and the clinical team—as well as those we serve—than a fully empowered and engaged professional community that creates the foundations and conditions for excellence for the foreseeable future.

Tim Porter-O'Grady, DM, EdD, ScD (h), APRN, FAAN
Senior Partner, Tim Porter-O'Grady Associates, Inc.
Atlanta, Georgia

Chapter 1

Introduction

The Concept Behind Shared Governance

> *With input from stakeholders inside and outside the organization,*
> *leaders are expected to shape agendas, not impose priorities;*
> *to allocate attention, not dictate results; and to define problems,*
> *not mandate solutions. These expectations we now have for leaders*
> *closely resemble conventional notions of governing.*
>
> —R. P. Chait, W. P. Ryan, and B. E. Taylor,
> Governance as Leadership

The increasing complexities of changes in healthcare have a growing number of institutions reexamining shared governance—a concept introduced into healthcare organizations in the 1970s—as an evidence-based method to support an empowering, integrated approach to healthcare services. Although there is no one "right" process model, the basic principles of shared governance are generic, viable, and measurable. This book takes some of the guesswork out of the various structures and processes behind shared governance. It provides strategies, case examples, and best practices to make the daily operations of shared governance meaningful and successful.

Quality, continual improvement, and excellence are embedded in healthcare practices across disciplines and services as the demand for value, safety, effectiveness, and efficiency grow and expand, directed at achieving outcomes that measure and increase the value of processes (i.e., shared governance). Therefore, this book also explores the relationship between shared governance and the American Nurses Credentialing Center (ANCC) Magnet Recognition Program® (MRP) as well as the International Organization for Standardization (ISO), and outlines the MRP and ISO expectations for shared governance practices.

What Is Shared Governance?

Before it can be solved, a problem must be clearly defined.
—William Feather

Shared governance has been referred to as a concept, a construct, a model, a system, a philosophy, and even as a movement. It is most often called shared decision-making or shared leadership in organizations that have implemented it. Universal principles and approaches engage the relationships and interactions needed to plan and design, implement, measure, and sustain shared governance in healthcare through an overlapping and integrating infrastructure (Porter-O'Grady, 2009).

Before going any further, then, an operational definition is needed to clarify this work and address the research and applications to practice that we find in shared governance.

Because shared governance reflects the mission, vision, and values of those who embrace it, it appears to be a fluid presence in each environment and practice setting. Over the years, many thought leaders, including Drs. Tim Porter-O'Grady and Robert Hess (coauthor of this book), have worked together to build autonomous interprofessional partners in healthcare through shared governance (see Appendix B for an extensive bibliography).

The *Random House Unabridged Dictionary* offers several definitions of the term *govern*, including: "to exercise in directing or restraining influence over; guide; the motives governing a decision; to have predominating influence." Building on that context, Hess' research in measuring shared governance developed and validated an 86-item instrument specifically designed to assess the six domains of shared governance in an organization and in the profession of nursing related to control, influence, authority, participation, access, and ability. Most instruments measure characteristics and some outcomes related to shared governance. However, the Index for Professional Governance (IPG) and the Index for Professional Nursing Governance (IPNG) have been researched and used to measure progress in developing and establishing shared governance in growing numbers of organizations. (See Chapter 6 for further details on the IPG and IPNG, and refer to Appendix A for the tools themselves.)

The management process model of shared governance and shared decision-making is based on the principles of partnership, equity, accountability, and ownership at the point of service. It empowers all members of the healthcare workforce to have a voice in decision-making. This facilitates diverse and creative input to advance the business and healthcare missions of the organization. In essence, this makes every employee feel like he or she is "part manager" with a personal stake in the success of the organization, which leads to:

- Longevity of employment
- Increased employee satisfaction

- Better safety and healthcare
- Greater patient satisfaction
- Shorter lengths of stay

Those who are happy in their jobs take greater ownership of their decisions and are more vested in patient outcomes. Employees, patients, the organization, and the surrounding communities all benefit from shared governance.

In effective shared governance, decision-making must be shared at the point of service to allow cost-effective service delivery and staff empowerment. This requires a decentralized management structure. Employee partnership, equity, accountability, and ownership occur at the point of service (e.g., on the patient care units) where at least 90% of the decisions need to be made.

The locus of control in the professional practice environment shifts to practitioners in matters of practice, quality, and competence. Only 10% of the decisions at the service or unit level belong to management (Porter-O'Grady and Hitchings, 2005).

Partnerships

Partnership links healthcare providers and patients along all points of service in the system; it is a collaborative relationship among all stakeholders and disciplines required for professional empowerment. Partnership is essential to building relationships, involves all staff members in decisions and processes, implies that each member has a key role in fulfilling the mission and purpose of the organization, and is critical to the effectiveness of the healthcare system (Porter-O'Grady and Hitchings, 2005).

Equity

Equity is the best method for integrating staff roles and relationships into structures and processes to achieve positive patient outcomes. Equity maintains a focus on services, patients, and staff; is the foundation and measure of value; and says that no role is more important than another. Although equity does not mean equality in terms of scope of practice, knowledge, authority, or responsibility, it does mean that each team member is essential in providing safe and effective care (Porter-O'Grady and Hitchings, 2005; Porter-O'Grady, Hawkins, and Parker, 1997).

Accountability

Accountability is a willingness to invest in decision-making and express ownership in those decisions. Accountability is the core of shared governance. It is often used interchangeably with responsibility and allows evaluation of role performance. It facilitates partnerships for sharing decisions and is secured in the roles by staff producing positive outcomes (Porter-O'Grady and Hitchings, 2005).

Ownership

Ownership is recognition and acceptance of the importance of everyone's work and that an organization's success is bound to how well individual staff members perform their jobs. Ownership designates where work is done and by whom to enable participation of all team members. It requires a commitment by each staff member for what is to be contributed, establishes a level of authority with an obligation to own what is done, and includes participation in devising purposes for the work (Koloroutis, 2004; Page, 2004; Porter-O'Grady and Hitchings, 2005). Shared governance activities may include participatory scheduling, joint staffing decisions, and shared service or unit responsibilities (e.g., every RN is trained to be in charge of his or her unit or area and shares that role with other professional team members, perhaps on a rotating schedule) to achieve the best patient care outcomes.

The old centralized management structures for command and control are ineffective for today's healthcare market, frequently inhibiting effective change and growth within the organization and limiting future market possibilities in recruitment and retention of qualified providers. Summative, hierarchical decision-making creates barriers to employee autonomy and empowerment. It can undermine service and quality of care. Today's patients are no longer satisfied with directive care. They, too, want partnership, equity, accountability, and mutual ownership in their own healthcare decisions and those of their family members (Institute of Medicine [IOM], 2011).Refer to Figure 1.1 for a look at the role of shared governance in these four points of service: partnership, equity, accountability, and ownership.

Interprofessional Shared Governance

Organizations are beginning to explore and integrate an interprofessional approach to shared governance, from clinical decisions at points of service to strategic priorities placed on complex issues by senior leadership (see Chapter 7). This approach often engages patients and families as partners. Keys to successful implementation of this approach to shared governance include active participation of all team members contributing to mutually respectful, trusting, collaborative, openly communicative, safe, and effective learning environments of care and practice across disciplines and departments. Interprofessional shared governance provides a unique structure for shared decision-making reflective of the current and evolving demands of an increasingly diverse and integrated care delivery system.

FIGURE 1.1 — Four characteristics of the principles of shared governance

PARTNERSHIP
- Role expectations negotiated
- Equality between players
- Relationship grounded in shared risk
- Clear expectations and contributions
- Establish solid measure of contribution to outcomes
- Defined horizontal linkages

EQUITY
- Each one's contributions are understood
- Payment reflects value of contribution to outcomes
- Role based on relationship, not status
- Team defines service roles, relationship, outcomes
- Team conflict and service issues defined by methodology
- Evaluation assesses team's outcomes and contributions

ACCOUNTABILITY
- Based on outcomes, not process
- Defined internally by person in role; embedded in roles
- Defines roles, not jobs; cannot be delegated
- Determined in advance of performance
- Performance validated by results
- Focus is on collective activities
- Self-described; dependent on and directly intersects with partnerships
- Shares evaluation
- Contributions-driven value
- Processes generally loud and noisy

OWNERSHIP
- All workers invested
- Every role and person has a stake in outcomes
- Rewards directly related to outcomes
- Every member associated with a team
- Relationships supported by processes
- Opportunity based on competence

Source: Porter-O'Grady, T. (2009c)

KEY PRINCIPLES
- Build on decisions and structure on a point-of-service foundation
- Always involve stakeholders in their own decisions
- Shared governance: an accountability-based approach, not a participative management model
- Team-based strategies are basic to structural design
- Locus of control placed wherever needed for decisions required
- Shared governance has no approval structures; it reflects relatedness between people and systems, not status within structures and systems
- Managers focus on context, staff on content
- Partnership, equity, accountability, ownership: undergirding principles of shared governance

History and Development of Shared Governance

The concepts of shared governance and shared decision-making are not new ones. Philosophy, education, religion, politics, business and management, and healthcare have all benefited from a variety of shared governance process models implemented in many diverse and creative ways across generations and cultures. For example:

- Socrates (470–399 BC), an ancient Greek philosopher, integrated shared governance concepts into his philosophies of education. The Socratic Method (answering a question with a question) calls for the teacher to facilitate the student's autonomous learning as the teacher guides him or her through a series of questions. The Socratic Method encourages students to use reason rather than appeal to authority.

- The government model for the United States was established on the concepts of shared governance—"of the people, by the people, for the people" (from Lincoln's Gettysburg Address, 1863)—wherein the very citizenry is directly responsible for the government on both state and federal levels. Political variations of this model of shared governance can also be seen in the European Union and the United Nations, where individual countries share in the decision-making on joint international matters.

- Eventually, shared governance found its way into the business and management literature (Laschinger, 1996; O'May and Buchan, 1999; Peters and Waterman, 1982). Organizations began to design formal structures and relationships around their leaders and employees. Positive outcomes emphasized movement from point of service outward. This differed from the more traditional, hierarchical method of moving from the organization downward in the previously used approach.

- In the late 1970s and early 1980s, shared governance found its way into the healthcare arenas as a form of participative management. It engaged self-managed work teams and grew out of the dissatisfaction nurses and other healthcare providers were experiencing with the institutions in which they practiced (McDonagh et al, 1989; O'May and Buchan, 1999; Porter-O'Grady, 1995).

The professional practice environment of healthcare has shifted dramatically over the past generation (American Association of Colleges of Nurses [AACN], 2002; American Organization of Nurse Executives [AONE], 2000; IOM, 2011). Rapid advances are occurring in:

- Biotechnology and cyberscience
- Disease prevention, patient safety, and management
- Relationship-based care
- Patients' roles in their own healthcare (i.e., active partners and not just passive recipients)

Economic constraints related to service reimbursement and corporatism have forced healthcare systems to cost-save by:

- Downsizing the professional workforce
- Changing staffing mixes
- Restructuring and reorganizing services
- Reducing support services for patient care
- Moving patients more rapidly to alternative care settings or discharge

Poor collaboration and ineffective communication among healthcare providers eventuate in sometimes devastating medical errors. The struggle to provide safe, quality care in the highly stressful—and sometimes highly charged—work environment today has resulted in limited success in recruitment and retention of qualified providers nationwide (AACN, 2002; Kohn, Corrigan, and Donaldson, 1999; Weinberg, 2003).

Shared Governance and Professional Practice Models

As economic realities continue to shift and change, so does practice. Tim Porter-O'Grady observed the following: "Reorganization in healthcare institutions is currently the rule rather than the exception. All healthcare participants are attempting to strategically position themselves in the marketplace" (1987, p. 281).

Developing an effective professional practice model for the economically constrained U.S. healthcare system is more important than ever. In the post–Affordable Care Act era, healthcare organizations are increasingly challenged to achieve positive outcomes, build workplace advocacy, and support recruitment as well as retention of the industry's shrinking workforce (Barden, 2009; IOM, 2011; Monaghan and Swihart, 2010; Porter-O'Grady and Malloch, 2010a; Swihart, 2011).

Mary K. Anthony (2004) describes some of the models that have evolved to provide structure and context for care delivery in the reshaping of professional practice:

- Those based on patient care assignment (i.e., working in teams)
- Accountability systems (i.e., primary care practice)
- Managed care (i.e., case management)
- Shared governance, based on professional autonomy and participatory, or shared, decision-making (i.e., relationship-based care)

Mary Koloroutis (2004) presents the integrated work of nurse leaders, researchers, and authors who have worked with a global community of healthcare organizations over the past 25 years. The result is a model for transforming practice that lends itself effectively to shared governance versus self-governance) in today's complex healthcare systems: relationship-based care (RBC). (See Figure 1.2 for a comparison of self-governance to shared governance.)

The RBC model embraces a philosophical foundation and operational framework for providing health services through relationships in a caring and healing environment that embodies the concepts of partnership, equity, accountability, and ownership in shared governance.

FIGURE 1.2 Self-governance vs. shared governance

Centralized Interactions (Self-Governance)	Decentralized Interactions (Shared Governance)
• Position-based • Distant from point of care/service • Hierarchical communication • Limited staff input • Separates responsibility/managers are accountable • We/they work environment • Divided goals/purpose • Independent activities/tasks	• Knowledge-based • Occurs at point of care/service • Direct communication • High staff input • Integrates equity, accountability, and authority for staff and managers • Synergistic work environment • Cohesive goals/purpose, ownership • Collegiality, collaboration, partnership

Shared decision-making occurs best in a decentralized organizational structure where those at the point of service are granted the autonomy and authority to make and determine the appropriateness of their own decisions. "When staff members are clear about their roles, responsibilities, authority, and accountability, they have greater confidence in their own judgments and are more willing to take ownership for decision-making at the point of care" (Koloroutis, 2004, p. 72). Decentralized decision-making is most successful when responsibility, authority, and accountability (R + A + A) are clearly delineated and assigned (Wright, 2002) in shared governance.

Responsibility

Responsibility is the clear and specific allocation of duties to achieve desired results. Assignment of responsibility is a two-way process. Responsibility is visibly given and visibly accepted. Acceptance is the essence of responsibility. However, individuals cannot accept responsibility without a level of authority.

Authority

Authority is the right to act and make decisions in the areas where one is given and accepts responsibility. When people are asked to share in the work, they must know their level of authority in which to carry out that work. Levels of authority must be given to those asked to take on responsibility. There are four levels of authority, or ways to be clear in communication and delegation of that authority (Wright, 2002):

- **Data gathering:** "Get information, bring it back to me, and I will decide what to do with it."
    - » **Example:** *Please go down and see if Mr. Jones has a headache and come back and tell me what he says.*

- **Data gathering + recommendations:** "Get the information (collect the data), look at the situation and make some recommendations, and I will pick from one of those recommendations what we will do next. I still decide."
    - » **Example:** *Please go down and see if Mr. Jones has a headache and come back and tell me what you would recommend that I give him.*

- **Data gathering + recommendations [pause] + act:** "Get the information (collect the data), look at the situation and make some recommendations, and pick one that you will do. But before you carry it out, I want you to stop (pause) and check with me before you do it." The pause is not necessarily for approval. It is more of a double-check to make sure everything was considered before proceeding.
    - » **Example:** *Please go down and see if Mr. Jones has a headache, come back and tell me what you would recommend for him, and then take care of him for me.*

- **Act and inform or update:** "Do what needs to be done and tell me what happened or update me later." There is no pause before the action.
    - » **Example:** *Please take care of Mr. Jones for me and update me on his status at the end of the shift.*

Accountability

Accountability begins when one reviews and reflects on his or her own actions and decisions, and culminates with a personal assessment that helps determine the best actions to take in the future.

For example, in shared governance, a manager or supervisor is accountable for patient care delivery in his or her area of responsibility. The manager or supervisor does not do all the tasks but does provide the resources employees need and ensures patient care delivery is done effectively by all staff members. In that patient care area, the manager or supervisor is accountable for setting the direction, looking at past decisions, and evaluating outcomes. Bedside providers and nurses, for example, are accountable for the overall care outcomes of assigned groups of patients for the time period they are there and for overseeing the big picture; however, other people (dietitians, therapists, pharmacists, laboratory technicians, and other healthcare providers) share in the responsibility for the subsequent tasks in meeting patients' needs.

Although definitions, models, structures, and principles of shared governance (sometimes called collaborative governance, participatory governance, shared or participatory leadership, staff empowerment, or clinical governance) vary, the outcomes are consistent. The evidence suggests that the benefits of implementation of shared governance and shared decision-making processes (detailed in Figure 1.3) can result in:

- Increased employee satisfaction with shared decision-making, related to increased responsibility combined with appropriate authority and accountability
- Increased professional autonomy with higher staff and manager or supervisor retention
- Greater patient and staff satisfaction
- Improved patient care outcomes
- Better financial states due to cost savings and cost reductions

Shared Governance and Relational Partnerships

The best [leader] is the one who has sense enough to pick
good [people] to do what he wants done, and self-restraint enough
to keep from meddling with them while they do it.

—*Theodore Roosevelt*

Professional nurses long ago identified shared governance as a key indicator of excellence in professional practice (McDonagh et al., 1989; Metcalf and Tate, 1995; Porter-O'Grady, 1987, 2001, 2004, 2009a, 2009b, 2009c). Tim Porter-O'Grady (2001) described shared governance as a management process model for providing a structure for organizing work within organizational settings. It allows strategies for empowering providers to express and manage their practice with a greater degree of professional autonomy. Personal and professional accountability are respected and supported within the organization. Leadership support for point-of-service staff enables them to maintain quality practice, job satisfaction, and financial viability when partnership, equity, accountability, and ownership are in place (Anthony, 2004; Green and Jordan, 2002; Koloroutis, 2004; Page, 2004; Porter-O'Grady, 2003a, 2003b; Porter-O'Grady and Malloch, 2010a, 2010b, 2010c).

Today's transformational relationship-based healthcare creates a new paradigm with different goals and objectives in organizational learning environments driven by technology. Leaders, administrators, and employees are learning and implementing new ways of providing care, new technologies, and new ways of thinking and working. In the process, they recognize more and more that the healthcare provider at the point of service is key to organizational success associated with changing the environments of care.

FIGURE 1.3	Benefits and challenges of shared governance	
Targets	Benefits	Challenges
For the patients, clients		
• Reduced mortality • Reduced morbidity • Increased patient and client satisfaction • Increased safety • Decreased "failure to rescue"	• Increased confidence in healthcare providers • Reduced confusion or concern about care due to increased collaboration among providers • Decreased lengths of stay	• Appropriate delegation of authority, roles, and responsibilities for care • Willingness by providers and managers to share authority for decision-making at points of service
For organizations		
• Decreased length of stay • Decreased cost of staff replacement • Increased opportunity to market institution • Variable costs of implementation	• Increased retention of experienced care providers • Anticipatory change • Broad-based horizontal relationships among systems • Balance between service accountability and system accountability • Fewer levels of management • Involved stakeholders, e.g., for resource-based decisions • Decisions reflect organizational mission, priorities, and goals	• Resources (fiscal, human, and material) for sustained shared governance • Resistance of managers to support staff through shared leadership (i.e., shared authority) • Obstacles to autonomous point-of-service decision-making that may exist within the organization • Transfer of influence and control away from senior and middle managers alone to include point-of-service staff
For healthcare providers		
• Lower turnover • Lower vacancy rates • Lower burnout rates • Lower emotional exhaustion • Decreased work-related injuries • Better interprofessional relationships • Higher employee satisfaction • Higher healthcare provider-to-patient ratio • Decreased medical errors	• Increased professionalism and accountability • Interdependent relationships among healthcare providers • Shared accountability, ownership, equity, and engaged partnerships • Increased collaboration and collegiality related to mutual trust, respect, and shared decision-making • Increased control over practice and decision-making related to competence, quality, safety, service, and practice	• Training and development of councils and council participants • Release from routine duties to participate in councils • Seeing shared governance as a "nurses only" process that does not impact fiscal or clinical activities or outcomes for other providers • Confusion about roles and responsibilities associated with shared governance

Health providers, managers and supervisors, interprofessional partners, and organizational leaders must be prepared for new roles, relationships, and ways of managing. Shared governance is about moving from a traditional hierarchical model to a relational partnership model of practice, as shown in Figure 1.4.

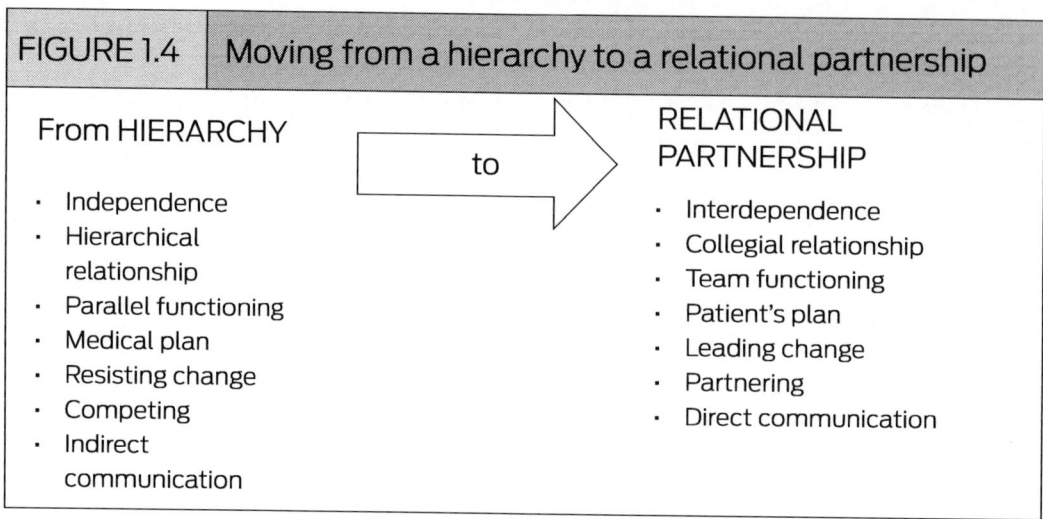

Successful relational partnerships in collaborative interprofessional practice (e.g., nurses, physicians, pharmacists, social workers, therapists) and multidisciplinary team members (e.g., administration, support services, environmental services and housekeeping) practice require understanding the roles of each partner. If the partners are not aware of what each brings to that relationship, they will have considerable problems collaborating, acting responsibly, and being accountable for decisions and care. Therefore, relational partnerships can be a complex and challenging framework for the shared governance professional practice model (Green and Jordan, 2004; Porter-O'Grady and Hitchings, 2005; Porter-O'Grady and Malloch, 2010a).

The key provider at points of service moves from the bottom to the center of the organization, becoming the only one who matters in a service-based organization—the one providing the care. Frontline employees who do the work connect the organization to the recipient of its service at the point of service. With this shift of focus, an entirely different sense and set of variables now affect the design of the organization. The paradigm at point of service has shifted to a relationship-based, staff-centered, patient-focused professional practice model of service in which managers or supervisors assume the role of servant leaders by managing resources and outcomes within the context of relational partnerships (Nightingale, 1992).

Patient-centered care

Patient-centered care differs from patient-focused care. The Institute for Healthcare Improvement (IHI) describes *patient-centered care* in the following way:

> Care that is truly patient-centered considers patients' cultural traditions, their personal preferences and values, their family situations, and their lifestyles. It makes the patient and their loved ones an integral part of the care team who collaborate with healthcare professionals in making clinical decisions. Patient-centered care puts responsibility for important aspects of self-care and monitoring in patients' hands—along with the tools and support they need to carry out that responsibility. Patient-centered care ensures that transitions between providers, departments, and healthcare settings are respectful, coordinated, and efficient. When care is patient-centered, unneeded and unwanted services can be reduced (2011).

IHI supports shared governance in recognizing the multifaceted challenges of advancing patient-centered care, and encourages organizations to identify best practices and systems changes in three areas:

1. Involving patients and families in the design of care
2. Reliably meeting patients' needs and preferences
3. Participating in informed shared decision-making

Healthcare research is guiding the development of initiatives for "reorganizing the delivery of healthcare services around what makes the most sense for patients" (IOM, 2001, 2011, p. 51). A few examples of patient-centered care initiatives include:

- Patient-centered medical homes
- Transforming care at the bedside (TCAB)
- Primary care (rather than specialty physician care)
- Midwives and birth centers
- Parish nursing
- Telehealth
- Community outreach (e.g., Program for All-Inclusive Care for Elders; *www.npaonline.org*)
- The transitional care model (IOM, 2011)

Patient-focused care refers to the caregiver's ability to focus his or her education, experience, and expertise on caring for the patient at the point of service and to facilitate organizational and community patient-centered care. To do this, caregivers must have managers or supervisors who are servant leaders, functioning differently in newly delineated roles (as agent or representative, advocate, ambassador, executor, intermediary, negotiator, proctor, promoter, steward, deputy, and emissary) and transforming practice settings in which patient-focused care occurs. Relational partnerships are built with equity, wherein the value of each of the participants is based on contributions to the relationship rather than on positions within the healthcare system.

Organizations must move to relational partnerships to be effective and sustain levels of excellence in service. Although frontline staff members are key to recruiting other employees, managers and supervisors are key to retaining them. Collateral and equity-based process models of shared governance define employees by the work they support in regard to each other rather than by their location or position in the system. For example, the manager or supervisor in the servant, or transformational, leader role provides human and material resources, support, encouragement, and boundaries for the employee in the service-provider role. Health providers, then, are accountable for key roles, decisions, and critical patient care outcomes around practice, quality, and competency.

Catalysts of change

Strong interprofessional collaborations with diverse professional perspectives based on variances in education, experience, and philosophy are essential to be successful in providing point-of-care services. For example:

- RNs bring a holistic (whole-istic) approach to care, managing diseases and disorders while considering psychosocial, spiritual, family, and community perspectives
- Pharmacists bring expertise in pharmacodynamics
- Physicians bring a more focused approach to diagnostically managing diseases and disorders with expertise in physiology, disease pathways, and treatments (IOM, 2011)

Shared governance as an organizational management process model for reshaping practice and decision-making requires a transformative shift. The resulting strategic change in organizational culture and leadership comes about through collaboration with interprofessional partners and multidisciplinary team members. Implementation demands a significant realignment in how leaders, employees, and systems transition into new relationships, responsibilities, and accountabilities. It begins with operationalizing the definitions and objectives, building relationships, and creating the design.

Chapter 2

Design a Structure to Support Shared Governance

The loftier the building,
the deeper must the foundation be laid.
—Thomas Kempis

Healthcare providers work closely with an ever-widening network of internal and external stakeholders and systems to meet the challenges of today's practice settings and provide safe, effective, quality care. They pull information from multiple sources to facilitate the interrelationships and collaborations among professionals and settings, and for care delivery within the larger organization and communities of practice.

Every model, structure, or process of shared governance looks different when appropriately implemented at each of these levels of the organization. The unique character of the organization, its mission, and its staff will yield a foundational organization management process model reflective of the depth and importance of practice and leadership contributions in that organization.

For example, providers collaborate with several departments for related services (e.g., mesosystems such as pharmacy and social services) prior to discharge when moving patients from the service or unit (the *microsystem*) through the organization and into the larger health system (the *macrosystem*). (See a description of these systems in Figure 2.1 and an illustration of a sample model in Figure 2.2.)

FIGURE 2.1	Systems descriptions	
ORGANIZATION LEVEL	DESCRIPTION	TEAMS
Health system macrosystem	Whole organization; communities of practice; teams focus on systems, strategic planning, resources allocations (human, material, and fiscal), professional governance, and relationships within the whole organization and communities of practice at local, national, and global levels	Health services; senior leaders: CEO, chief operations officer, chief financial officer, chief marketing officer, chief nursing officer, chief information officer; internal and external stakeholders
Facility (departments or divisions) mesosystem	Major divisions and systems; teams focus on systems and relationships, the structure, framework, and context that support the team's activities (e.g., shared governance, risk management, quality systems, human resources, fiscal services); teams build and sustain professional relationships, interactions, and connections among team members, other teams, and the services they provide to achieve clinical and service-related outcomes	Nursing, medicine, pharmacy, social services, dietetics, laboratory services, environmental management services, radiology, physical and occupational health, rehabilitation, surgery, critical care, informatics, women's health, nursery, pediatrics, and other clinical and departmental service lines
Clinical (unit council) microsystem	Frontline service units; smaller functional units and teams who focus on specific functions and activities that are the work of the organization at the points of service or care; work collaboratively to facilitate, improve, and advance relationships and services provided by the multidisciplinary team members and interprofessional partners	Nurses, managers and supervisors, social services and social workers, pharmacists, physicians, clinical nurse leaders, case managers, clinical specialists, educators and staff development specialists, chaplains and clinical spiritual leaders and pastors, risk managers, and others, including patients and families

© 2014 HCPro

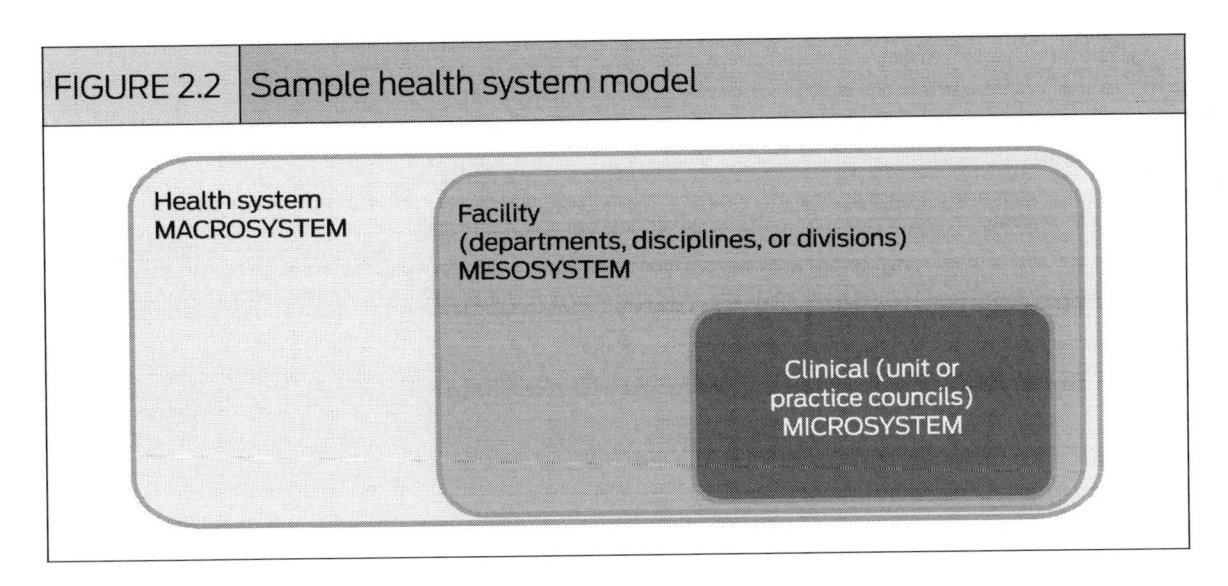

FIGURE 2.2 | Sample health system model

Health system MACROSYSTEM

Facility (departments, disciplines, or divisions) MESOSYSTEM

Clinical (unit or practice councils) MICROSYSTEM

Many features of shared governance are similar enough to provide guidance in designing a structure that will support it in practice (see Figures 2.3 and 2.4, Porter-O'Grady, 2004, 2009c). (See Appendix B in the back of this book for many other excellent resources for designing and implementing a shared governance organization management process model.)

Common Characteristics of Shared Governance Structures

All shared governance structures have the following characteristics and features in common (see Appendix 3 for a detailed comparison):

- There is no one way to design or structure a shared governance management process model.
- Shared governance is grounded in practice at the practice or unit (microsystem) level.
- Staff members are responsible, accountable, and have authority over all decisions related to professional practice (practice, quality, and competence).
- Frontline staff members are elected to the positions they hold in the shared governance structure by their peers rather than appointed by management.
- Shared governance needs to be implemented service- or departmentwide at the mesosystem level rather than unit by unit or practice at the microsystem level, thereby creating silos.
- Management cannot remove an elected staff representative except as an official action against the employee (e.g., substandard work performance, unethical conduct, failure to perform assigned duties related to job description).

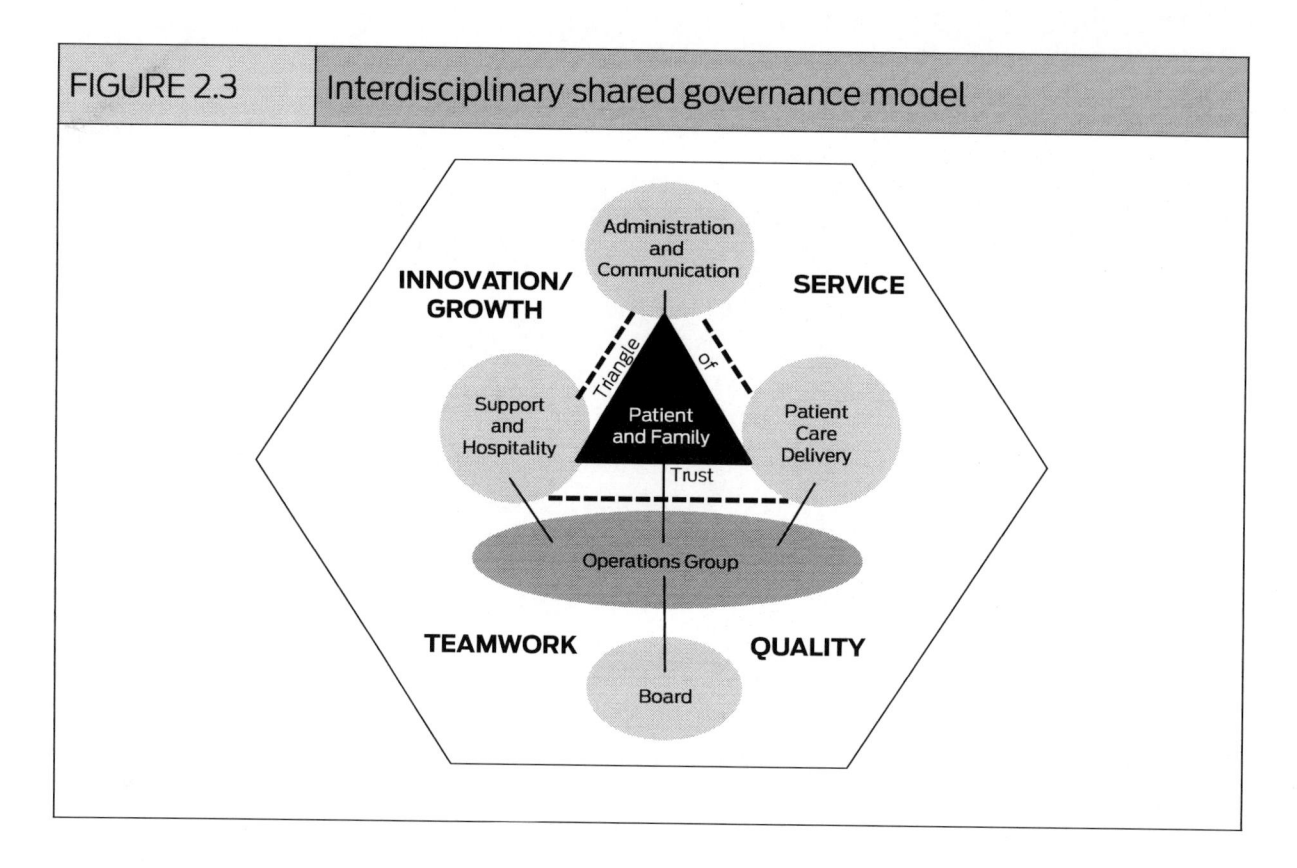

FIGURE 2.3   Interdisciplinary shared governance model

Diagram: A hexagon labeled with INNOVATION/GROWTH, SERVICE, TEAMWORK, and QUALITY at its corners. Inside is a "Triangle of Trust" with Administration and Communication at the top, Support and Hospitality at the left, and Patient Care Delivery at the right, surrounding Patient and Family in the center. Below are the Operations Group and the Board.

- Practice- or unit-level operational processes are defined by frontline staff.

- Direct-care providers drive the structuring of the shared governance process.

- Management, in the servant leader role, provides the support, encouragement, resources (financial, human, and material), training, and boundaries (organizational and management) necessary for success.

- A coordinating group composed of staff and management provides guidance about issues affecting the department or discipline, communicating the organization's strategic plan, developing shared governance bylaws, approving departmental or service expenditures or budgets, and helping determine accountabilities for appropriate groups and members within the shared governance structure.

- Shared governance is driven by bylaws or rules, however, some practices or units will use project charters instead of bylaws. In current usage among many healthcare organizations, a charter is essentially a description of the scope, purpose, and objectives, and participation guidelines for

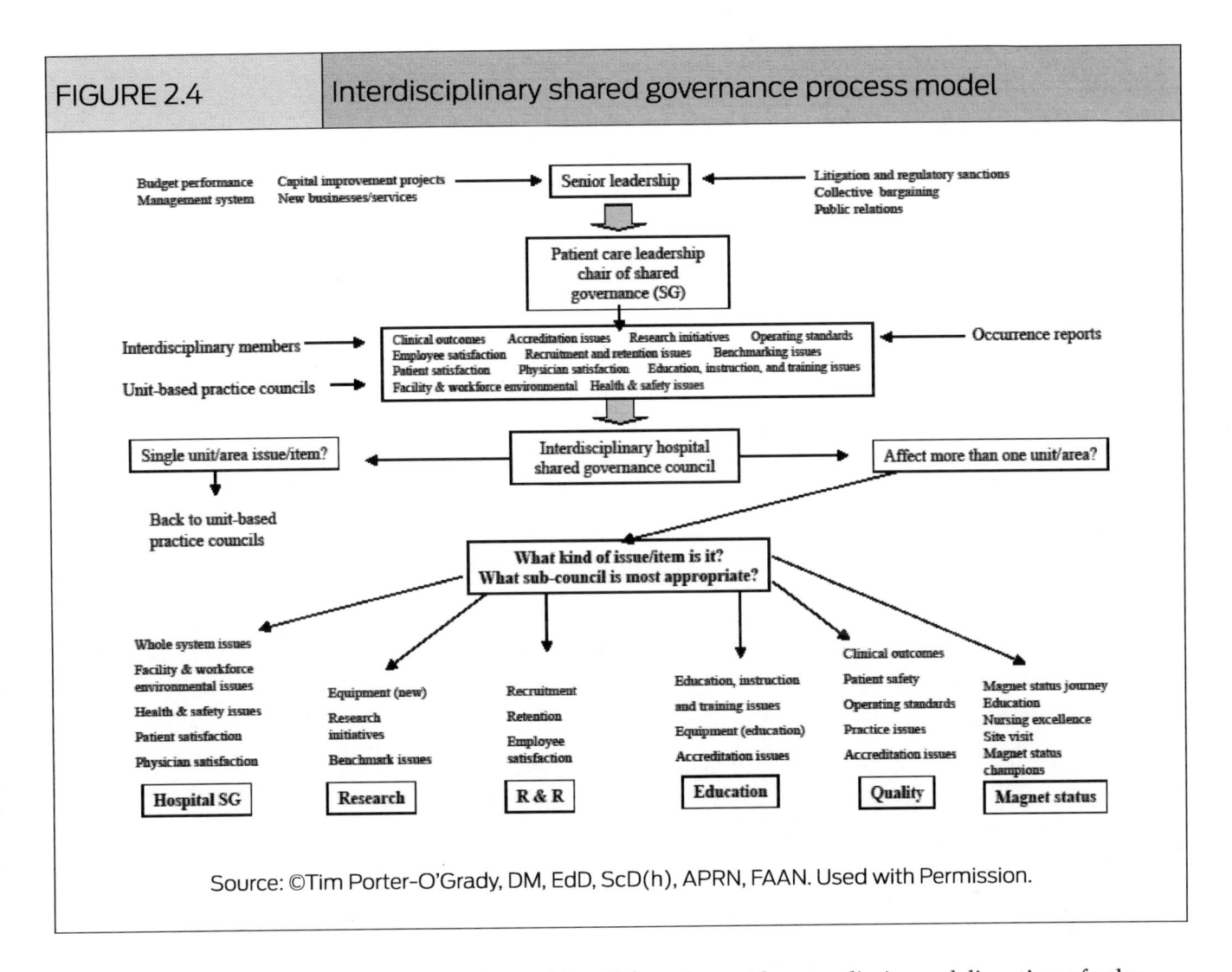

FIGURE 2.4 — Interdisciplinary shared governance process model

Source: ©Tim Porter-O'Grady, DM, EdD, ScD(h), APRN, FAAN. Used with Permission.

a committee or council. The charter identifies and provides a preliminary delineation of roles and responsibilities of participants and stakeholders, defines the authority and duties of the leadership, and serves as a reference of authority for the committee or council. Though similar to bylaws in many ways, a charter is usually considered to be a more flexible, less formal set of rules, with voting often by consensus, and rarely incorporates parliamentary procedure.

- Shared governance is responsibility- and accountability-based, defined by what employees do, how they do it, and the outcomes expected from practice at point of service (see Figure 2.5 for the characteristics of accountability and responsibility).

FIGURE 2.5	Characteristics of accountability and responsibility
ACCOUNTABILITY	RESPONSIBILITY
• Defined by outcomes, not process • Self-described • Embedded in roles • Dependent on partnerships • Shares evaluation • Contributions-driven value	• Defined by functions, not outcomes • Delegated • Specific tasks and routines dictated • Isolative • Supervisor evaluation • Tasks-driven value

Shared governance has a primary focus. It is a process with core principles. Effective shared governance engages constant assessment and evaluation to be flexible and adaptive to accomplish the following:

- Transform the organization into a practice model of shared decision-making in a decentralized relational partnership with individual professional responsibility, accountability, and authority over practice decisions at points of service
- Empower the staff in unexpected ways, such as nontraditional involvement in operations and decision-making
- Shift some of the accountability historically part of the management or supervisory role or owned by the organization to direct-care providers
- Involve many participants who, through shared decision-making, undertake multiple essential roles that are mutual in their exercise and on which each partner depends
- When implemented effectively, shared governance affects the organization as a whole, divisionwide and at practice and unit levels

Basic Requirements of All Shared Governance Systems

Four elements are essential to the successful implementation of shared governance in the earliest stages of process development. A *steering group* (or design team) is critical to ensure these elements are in place for designing and implementing a successful shared governance process. Following implementation, the steering group often evolves into a coordinating (or operations) council to continue to move the work toward sustainment.

The four essential elements are:

1. A *committed executive* must be invested in process empowerment and willing to undertake the efforts and energy necessary to implement shared governance.
2. A *strong management team* is essential in terms of commitment to one another, to providers, to the organization, and to building the structure and implementing the process.

3. *Employees* who have gained a basic understanding of shared governance and can build on that understanding with a working knowledge of what is to be accomplished. There must be a clear destination.
4. *A plan and a timeline for implementation,* both of which are critical for benchmarking and charting progress points.

Guidelines for forming the governance bodies include the following:
- Create a decision-making group that is empowered to make decisions that form a baseline for thinking organizationally when implementing shared governance.
- Designate an appropriately sized group (usually seven to 10 participants and generally no more than 14 to 15) to facilitate effective group decision-making. It generally requires about seven people to represent the organization or service line (e.g., nursing, social services, pharmacy, and medicine) equitably. NOTE: The presence of more than 15 participants reduces the group's ability to reach consensus and move the agenda and work forward.
- Ensure that decisional groups are accountability-based.
- Within the organization, all groups, committees, and task forces relate to governance bodies or central councils.
- Communication within and across all groups, committees, task forces/teams, and governing or central councils is critical to the success of implementation and ongoing operations of the shared governance management process model.

Basic Structural Process Models of Shared Governance

Four basic structural models of shared governance have emerged in America in the past 40 years (Anthony, 2004; Green and Jordon, 2004; Porter-O'Grady, 1986, 1987, 1991, 2009c; Porter-O'Grady and Hitchings, 2005; Swihart, 2011): (1) congressional, (2) councilor, (3) administrative, and (4) unit- or practice-level. All four models are based on essentially the same principles but reflect differing specific characteristics depending on the intention of the model, the design and structure of the organization, and the services building it.

Congressional model of shared governance

One of the first models developed for shared governance, the congressional model reflects primarily a specific practice orientation in its design. This model features a staff congress composed of an elected president and a cabinet or senate of officers and all of the professional staff who oversee the operations of a unit, area, practice, or department (including management and point-of-service employees). The various committees of the congress, who are delegated by the congress to make certain decisions and to have certain powers, are selected out of that congress and report back to the cabinet or senate. The congress defines its accountabilities and assigns those accountabilities its various committees.

FIGURE 2.6 The congressional model of shared governance

```
Management & Executives
    |
Cabinet —or— Senate
    |
P  QA  E  R  M
Committees of Congress
Staff Congress
```

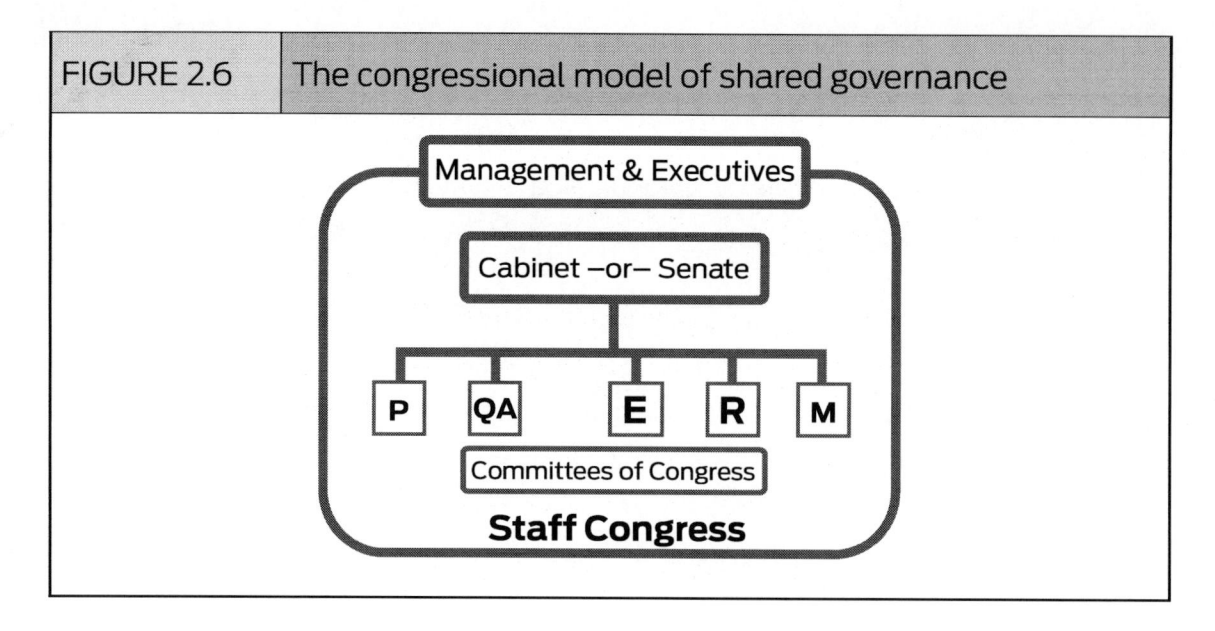

Five basic accountabilities emerge from the committees of congress, as shown in the Figure 2.6 diagram of the congressional model (adapted from Porter-O'Grady, 1991):

1. Practice (P)
2. Quality management (QA)
3. Professional development and education (E)
4. Research (R)
5. Management or leadership (M)

These accountabilities reflect the basic professional accountabilities of the disciplines. The work of the organization is carried out in the committees of congress and disseminated to direct-care employees and other stakeholders from there.

Councilor model of shared governance

The councilor model is very similar to the congressional model and is one of the most commonly used models in healthcare. It consists of councils on clinical practice, quality assurance, management, research, advocacy, and staff development and education. The term *council* is used to differentiate the work of the shared governance organizational management process teams from the committees and task groups, which are usually groups of people chosen or appointed to perform a specified service or function. For example, all unit- or practice-level decisions related to professional practice, quality, and competence are given over to a unit or practice council. However, inquiries and decisions relative to policies and procedures are given over to the standards of care committee.

The councils are empowered by the staff to perform the basic accountabilities identified in the congressional model: practice, quality management, research, staff development and education, and management. However, the structure is slightly different. Councils are empowered with the authority rather than the congress. Each council is delegated by the organization with accountability and authority for decisions that fall within the context of that council. For example, all practice decisions belong to the practice council, all quality management decisions belong to the quality council, and so on.

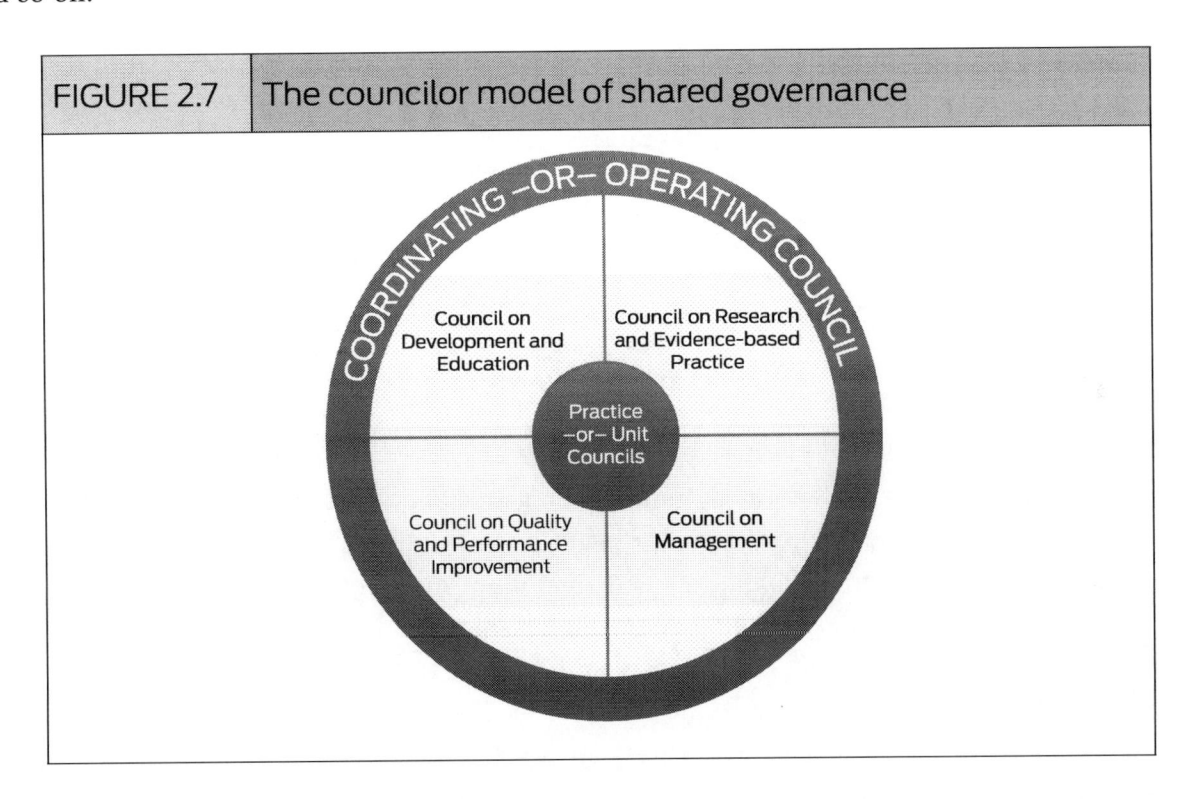

FIGURE 2.7 The councilor model of shared governance

Coordinating –or– Operating Council
- Council on Development and Education
- Council on Research and Evidence-based Practice
- Council on Quality and Performance Improvement
- Council on Management

Center: Practice –or– Unit Councils

With the exception of the management council and the research council, all councils are made up predominantly of direct-care staff. Direct-care staff members make up about 90% of the councils and make the decisions related to accountabilities for practice, quality, and competency that are staff-based. In that way, actual accountability shifts from the traditional management framework to a staff framework as determined by the locus of control or the legitimate place of that accountability. For example, practice should always be in the hands of the practitioners; therefore, practice decisions are undertaken by practicing clinicians who are at the point of service or care. Responsibility, authority, and accountability for those decisions, policies, and outcomes rest with them. See Figure 2.7 for a diagram of the councilor model (adapted from Porter-O'Grady, 1991).

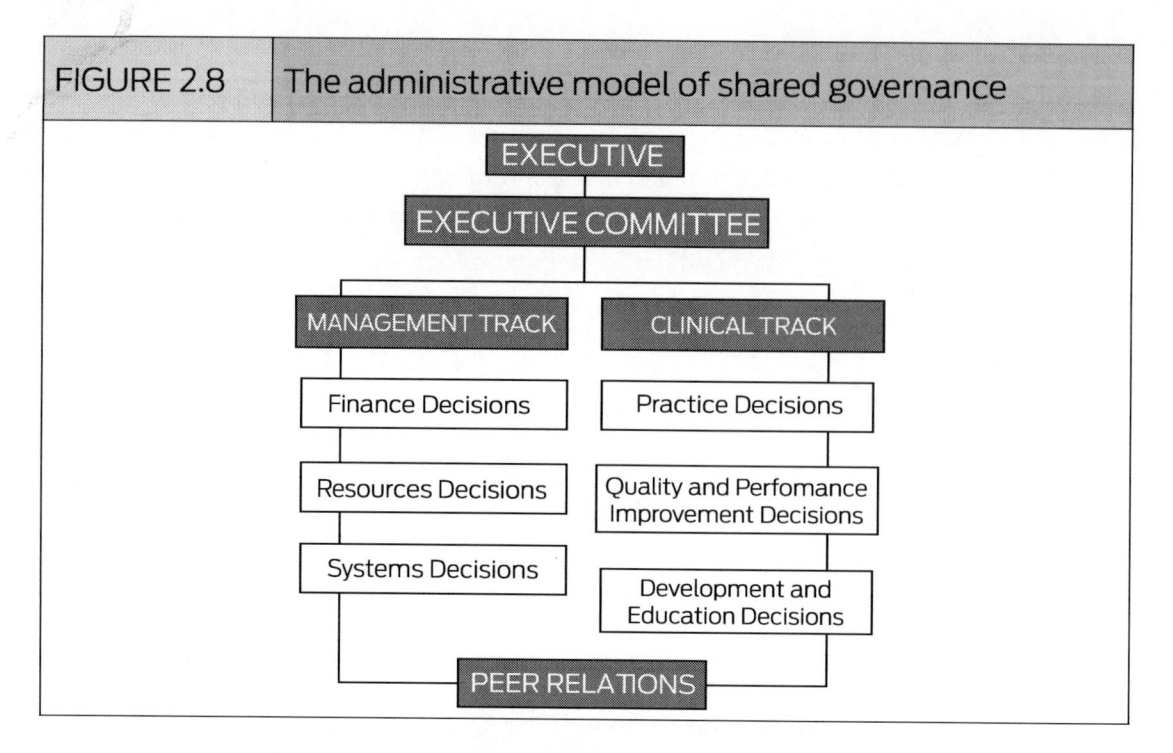

FIGURE 2.8 — The administrative model of shared governance

```
                        EXECUTIVE
                   EXECUTIVE COMMITTEE
                    /                \
         MANAGEMENT TRACK        CLINICAL TRACK
                |                      |
         Finance Decisions      Practice Decisions
                |                      |
         Resources Decisions    Quality and Performance
                |               Improvement Decisions
         Systems Decisions             |
                |               Development and
                |               Education Decisions
                        PEER RELATIONS
```

Administrative model of shared governance

The administrative model follows more traditional organizational lines of management and practice, with each having separate groups that address specific functions and accountabilities. This model resembles a traditional hierarchy with two structural units, management and clinical. These structural units are generally aligned in a top-down relationship, although both tracks may evolve to include both managers and staff as implementation advances. All work is done by committees and reported back to the overarching council or committee. The executive committee may make decisions on information provided for all clinical issues that concern more than one committee along either or both tracks. See Figure 2.8 for a diagram of the administrative model (adapted from Hess, 2009, and Porter-O'Grady, 1991).

The structural familiarity in communicating decisions upward is a key characteristic of this model. Decision-making groups within an administrative model are composed of at least 50% staff or a representative proportion of staff to management depending on the degree of organizational commitment to direct-care providers' participation in shared governance.

Practice- or unit-level model of shared governance

The practice- or unit-level model is rarely used. (NOTE: This is a structural model and is not to be confused with the practice- or unit-level councils in the councilor model.) The design principles are similar but the structure is fundamentally different. The culture of the practice or unit gives it form. Members define their own basic accountabilities; practices or units become entities unto themselves and make decisions about what they do and how they do it that may not impact the organization outside of the practice or unit.

One of the problems with this model might be an individual, insular, cultural application of shared governance with no integrating or coordinating principles from the division or department as a whole giving it guidance. Individual practices or units may build powerful decision-making models that direct-care providers exemplify and appreciate but may operate to jeopardize the structures of the whole division, service, or organization. However, the accountabilities defined in this model do work well when adapted to the councilor model for practice- or unit-level councils working in tandem, or in partnership, with the meso- and macrosystems of the organization. See Figure 2.9 for a diagram of a practice- or unit-level model of shared governance (adapted from Hess, 2009; Porter-O'Grady, 1991, 2009c; Swihart, 2011), and refer to Appendix 28 for a useful unit or practice council worksheet).

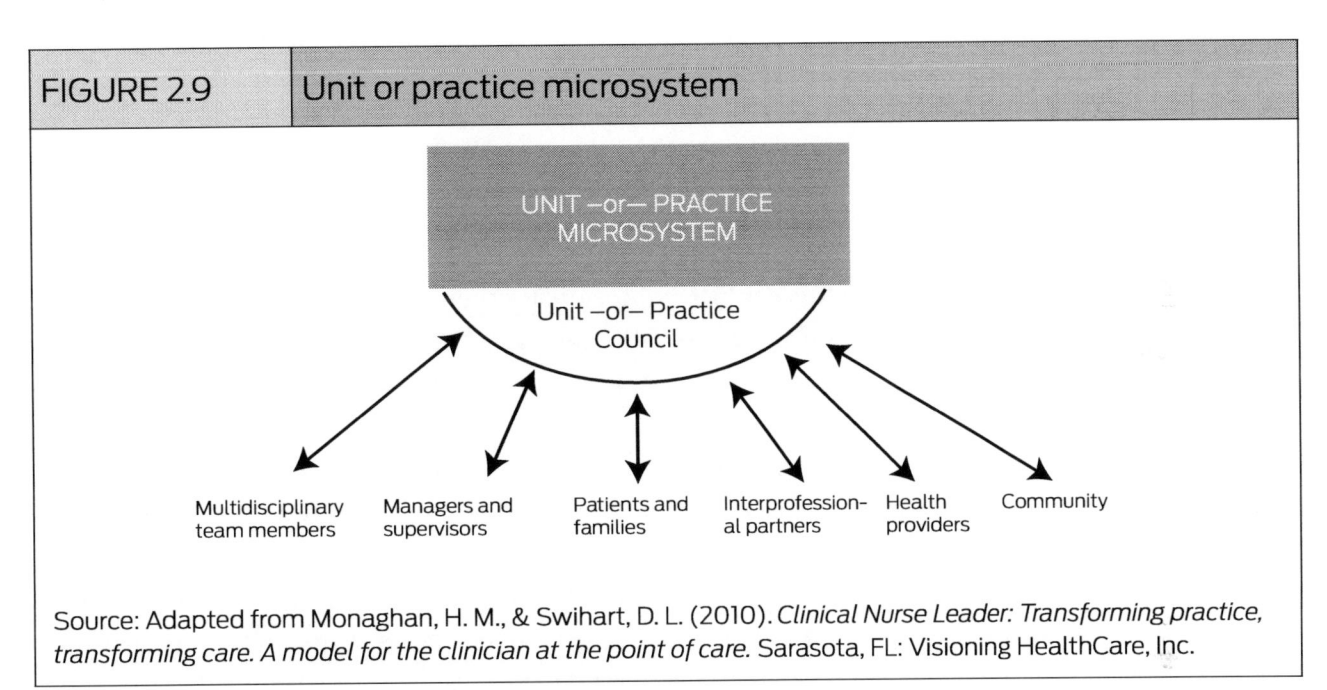

FIGURE 2.9 — Unit or practice microsystem

UNIT —or— PRACTICE MICROSYSTEM

Unit —or— Practice Council

- Multidisciplinary team members
- Managers and supervisors
- Patients and families
- Interprofessional partners
- Health providers
- Community

Source: Adapted from Monaghan, H. M., & Swihart, D. L. (2010). *Clinical Nurse Leader: Transforming practice, transforming care. A model for the clinician at the point of care.* Sarasota, FL: Visioning HealthCare, Inc.

Best practice in autonomous practice through unit councils

Contributing author: Solimar Figueroa, MSN, MHA, BSN, RN, CNOR, Miami, Florida

Baptist Health South Florida piloted implementation of autonomous direct-care nurse unit-level competency assessments on a medical-surgical unit utilizing their unit councils (i.e., unit practice councils [UPC]). They chose to adapt Wright's model (2005) and Swihart's Competency Decision Worksheet (see Appendix 5) for the pilot. Previously, competency validations had been done through biannual skills fairs. Attendance in these skills fairs was mandated for compliance.

The Wright model was presented to unit staff at the UPC monthly meeting. They were provided definitions and descriptions of the following:

- Competency assessment, purpose, and benefits
- Roles and delineation of internal and external stakeholders

- Processes involved in the transition to this approach for competency validation
- Selecting unit-level competencies based on what is new, changed, problematic, and/or high-risk and time-sensitive
- Training staff in peer verification, monitoring processes and activities, and reporting structures for outcomes

The proposal for implementation of unit-level competency validations reflected an organizational culture shift. The newly delineated roles of the stakeholders for the pilot involving the manager, nurse clinicians, and point-of-care staff were clearly and distinctly articulated to facilitate more successful outcomes. The unit-level competency model promoted accountability and best practices through the active engagement of the UPC members and direct-care nurses.

The UPC members disseminated the information presented to the council to the rest of the staff by following "trees" of communication. Each UPC member has a corresponding tree with between five and 10 assigned staff members. The staff received information from the UPC and then communicated back through their UPC representatives which competencies they identified as important for them. The unit council collected the information, and UPC members selected the competencies for the unit and determined the duration of each competency cycle (e.g., once, ongoing, annually, quarterly).

The collaboration among the manager, staff, and nurse clinicians in establishing the unit-level competencies was a phenomenal success based on the reported unit outcomes from the pilot. For example, the peer verification process embedded in the Wright model empowered the nurses to take charge of their professional practice. Nurses were trained on how to give reflective feedback to their colleagues as they selected and validated identified competencies at the unit level. This collegial, peer-to-peer approach promoted better communication among staff, encouraging them to help one another during the selection of competencies and validation processes. This gives the staff more autonomy in their own professional practice, competence, and quality, which contributes to improved patient care outcomes, satisfaction, safety, and compliance. It is one of the many best practices found at Baptist Health South Florida.

Shared governance demands an investment of effort and time by all partners from all levels of the healthcare system. As providers reshape and transform the professional practice community, the necessity for a relational partnership between management and direct-care providers in decision-making affects the design and structuring of service in the professional practice environment. In the process, knowledge of the basic concepts and a commitment to them is a prerequisite to the design and implementation processes.

Chapter 3

Build a Structure to Support Shared Governance

If the infrastructure does not consciously bring the teams together on an ongoing basis to build their relationships and to integrate their practice, partnerships will not be created, and the duplication, repetition, and fragmentation of care will not stop.
—Bonnie Wesorick

In Chapters 1 and 2, we gained a basic understanding of the concept behind shared governance and were introduced to some more common structural process models that complement the fundamental requirements of all shared governance systems. To be successful in creating a structure to support shared governance, you will need strategic planning, a representative design team (or redesign team, a steering group), and active, empowered engagement of interprofessional partners, leadership, multidisciplinary team members, and frontline staff.

In this chapter, we will look at how to implement shared governance, discuss how to lead strategic change, explore perspectives and formats of various shared governance models and systems, consider bylaws, articles, and charters, and identify a number of tips and tools along the way to help you. Let's begin.

Part 1. Implementing Shared Governance

The greatest amount of wasted time is the time not getting started.
—Dawson Trotman

Venner Farley observed, "For nurses, restructuring means change . . . Nurses must have a great capacity for change in order to accept the challenges of creating our future. The rewards will be substantial: autonomy and independence within a framework of collaboration and colleagueship." She encouraged providers to begin thinking and behaving differently as they embrace change along five parameters (2000):

- Face reality as it is
- Be open and honest with everyone
- Don't manage . . . *lead*
- Change before you have to
- Recognize that [providers] must seek and maintain a competitive advantage

Part 2. Leading Strategic Change

One of the reasons people don't achieve their dreams is that they desire to change their results without changing their thinking.
—John C. Maxwell

The changes in pace, demand, technological complexity, and patient populations today are greater than ever before. Consequently, the costs of resistance to those changes and failure to implement collaborative partnerships in shared decision-making can be catastrophic.

Healthcare providers have choices about where and how they will work. They are no longer willing to work for authoritarian top-down management systems. Nurses and physicians, among others, are choosing American Nurses Credentialing Center (ANCC) Magnet Recognition Program® (MRP) hospitals with high-involvement shared governance structures and processes and evolving professional practice models. Strategic changes related to implementation of shared governance include structural changes, organizational changes, cultural changes, and individual changes, such as those listed in Figure 3.1 (Porter-O'Grady, 2004).

A fundamental part of undertaking the processes associated with implementing shared governance and achieving successful outcomes is grounded in leading strategic change (Black and Gregersen, 2008), which becomes the driving force for defining and restructuring professional relationships. Every decision and action is set on some idea or theory that events or actions will result in predetermined outcomes. These are mental maps—beliefs about cause and effect—that guide people's decisions and behaviors. Most mental maps are forged in experience.

Changing mind maps

When people work successfully together in particular ways to make recurring decisions and complete repetitive tasks, they begin to assume these are the ways things should be done. This works well except when things change. Black and Gregersen (2008) offer insights for changing mind maps that

FIGURE 3.1	Strategic changes related to implementing shared governance
STRUCTURAL CHANGES	**INDIVIDUAL CHANGES**
• Multidisciplinary work flow patterns • Communication structures • Ongoing assessment of work patterns • Access to resources • Investment at all levels of the organization • Increasing dependence on interdependence • Role definitions and descriptions • Movement away from status determinations • Based on accountabilities, not hierarchies	• New realities • Degrees of change • Sound practice standards • Clear and strong ethics • Dialogue and communication • Honesty and integrity • Curiosity and creativity • Willingness to seek and abide by consensus (or majority vote, *e.g.*) • Able to express concerns and ideas • Structured risk-taking • Competency • Varying degrees of involvement • Increasing self-confidence
ORGANIZATIONAL CHANGES	**CULTURAL CHANGES**
• Salaried work roles • Reward systems; achievement rewards • Gain-sharing strategies • Role accountabilities clarification • Partnerships • Mentoring and precepting roles • Variable loci of leadership roles • Work design (staff driven) • Patient-centered care redesign • New orientation and socialization processes	• Reward systems altered • Continuous management development • Continuous leadership (manager and staff) development • Career enhancement programs • Hiring and termination processes • Staff role ownership, including position descriptions • Benefits programs • Unit and service programs vs. divisional ones

prevent people from changing and from maintaining the changes in place, one of the greatest obstacles to implementing shared governance in professional practice settings. Change the individual, and the organization will follow. Let's take a closer look what they discovered.

Change is not easy. It begins and ends with the mental maps about the organization and the jobs employees entertain in their heads. If those maps cannot be rewritten, if the brain barrier cannot be broken, there is nothing new for hearts and hands to follow. Without a compelling case for change, staff-centered, patient-focused, relationship-based care in shared decision-making will not follow.

Resistance to change is fundamental and biologically hardwired into humans. We are programmed for survival, to resist random change, and to maintain stability and sameness. Black and Gregersen (2008, p.3) call this the "map-hugging dynamic." Providers encountering shared governance for the first time may have difficulty letting go of old maps and ways of doing things.

The fundamental change process or cycle is based on the 80/20 principle, which says that 80% of the work comes from 20% of the workers. This explains why so many change initiatives fail: Only 20% of the employees capture 80% of the picture of strategic change. Black and Gregersen (2003, p. 13) identify four stages of successful strategic change:

- Stage 1: Do the right thing and do it well
- Stage 2: Discover that the right thing is now the wrong thing
- Stage 3: Do the new right thing, but do it poorly at first
- Stage 4: Eventually do the new right thing well

Leading strategic change in transforming professional practice through shared governance and the essentials of the principles identified in the ANCC MRP, for example, requires organizations to channel efforts in training, educating, and empowering others to get ahead of the change curve to master anticipatory change rather than subject themselves constantly to reactionary or crisis change (McClure and Hinshaw, 2002).

Brain barriers

So how exactly does remapping change work? Black and Gregersen (2008) discuss three primary brain barriers leading to failed change and the keys to successfully overcoming those barriers and delivering strategic change in healthy organizations.

1. **Barrier:** Failure to see the need for change when what they have already been doing seems to still be working for them.
   - *Key for success: Contrast.* Look at key contrasts in how strategies, structures, cultural values, processes, technologies, practice models, and approaches to leadership that worked in the past are no longer effective in the present or appropriate for the future.
   - *Key for success: Confrontation.* Leaders may have to confront employees with clear and compelling evidence between past, present, and future contrasts to help them see before they can move to change. They cannot—they will not—change if they do not see a need to do so.

2. **Barrier:** Failure to move after they see the need to change because they do not believe in the new path, their ability to walk it, or the rewarding outcomes of the journey and destination.

- *Key for success: Destinations.* Make sure everyone sees the destination clearly to gain belief in the move to shared governance. People cannot change if they do not see the destination clearly or understand where they are going.
- *Key for success: Resources.* Give them the skills, resources, and tools they need to reach the destination and participate in shared governance.
- *Key for success: Rewards.* Deliver valuable rewards along the journey that have meaning to the employee. People value many things. The ARCTIC assessment tool (see Figure 3.2) can help identify rewards that would have greater meaning to people and more power to move change and successfully implement shared governance (adapted from Black and Gregersen, 2008, p. 84).

3. **Barrier:** Failure to finish because they are tired and lost.
    - *Key for success: Champions.* Trained and motivated change champions are needed close to the action in every practice setting from the moment that the decision to change is implemented.
    - *Key for success: Charting.* Progress must be measured at all levels in the organization and reported. Performance—good, bad, or indifferent—needs to be communicated to staff members. Successful change requires monitoring and communicating at the individual level.

FIGURE 3.2	ARCTIC assessment tool
ARCTIC	Rewards
ACHIEVEMENT	• Accomplishment: need to meet or beat goals, to do better in the future than one has done in the past • Competition: need to compare one's performance with that of others and do better than others do
RELATIONS	• Approval: need to be appreciated and recognized by others • Belonging: need to feel a part of and accepted by the group
CONCEPTUAL THINKING	• Problem solving: need to confront problems and create answers • Coordination: need to relate pieces and integrate them into a whole
IMPROVEMENT	• Growth: need to feel continued improvement and growth as a person, not just improved results • Exploration: need to move into unknown territory for discovery
CONTROL	• Competence: need to feel personally capable and competent • Influence: need to influence others' opinions and actions

Leading strategic change by breaking the three brain barriers involves remapping old behaviors and guiding staff through the process individually first to ultimately impact the organization as a whole. Failure to see is a problem of entrenched, successful maps; high contrast and confrontation is needed to break through this barrier. Failure to move happens when smart people resist going from doing the wrong thing well to doing the right new thing poorly. It takes ensuring that the destination is clear, resources are in place, and valued rewards are provided to break through this barrier. Finally, failure to finish is a consequence of staff members getting tired and lost. Therefore, they do not go fast enough or far enough. Champions and open communication about progress, good or bad, is critical for breaking through this barrier.

Change is constant. It is the only real absolute in healthcare. Shared governance cannot be successful until all partners come together on how to lead strategic change. Dr. Michael Peterman (2011), an organizational development psychologist and change management architect, recommends that once the barriers to leading strategic change are understood, organizations should use a change management team to:

- Develop a vision and strategy for change
- Design and manage the change process
- Guide execution of the strategy
- Make the case for change
- Build motivation to change
- Enable and support change
- Anticipate and address sources of resistance (e.g., what are the organizational and individual forces opposing and supporting change leading to successful implementation)
- Reinforce and anchor change
- Provide accurate and timely communication

Making the case for change

Why should I change? *Why* before how ... Make a compelling case—the most important part of any major change—and teach representatives from each practice or unit council how to present it. Peterman (2011) describes components for building a compelling case for change:

- Ask if change is dependent on having a viable solution to the questions
- Describe why the change is a viable solution to the problem at hand
- Describe the nature of the change (i.e., the vision)
- Explain why the change is necessary
- Identify the benefits of change

- Anticipate and address sources of resistance
- Make presentations specific to target audience
- Incorporate feedback from key stakeholders
- Use a credible presenter to deliver the case for change
- Connect shared governance to what people value
- Include feedback from internal and external stakeholders at all levels
- Make sure the message has emotional appeal
- Use tools like metaphors, storytelling and exemplars, and case studies
- Include supporting data
- Communicate the case for change effectively and repeatedly

In the absence of a compelling case for change, motivation will likely be insufficient. Once the case for change has been made and accepted, it is time to move forward with the design, establishment, and maturing of shared governance structures and processes.

Part 3. Shared Governance Systems

Perspective and format

The ultimate measure of a man is not where he stands
in moments of comfort and convenience, but where he stands
at times of challenge and controversy.
　　　　　—Dr. Martin Luther King, Jr.

Structure your shared governance format and vision carefully. Identify organizational and service purposes, objectives, goals, direction, and strategic plans; reflect the organization's mission; and determine the roles providers and service leaders will have in shared governance: conceptual base, philosophy, objectives, care standards, performance measures, quality management and performance improvement, professional development, and practice.

Designing the shared governance process

Select members from each service, discipline, and multidisciplinary team to form a shared governance design team (or forum, group, steering committee, or coordinating group). They will obtain feedback from leadership and staff; consider providers' objectives and the organization's goals, mission, and philosophy; and draft a process model for shared governance. The final design will be selected by staff and leadership to represent an integrated process and structure for shared decision-making toward positive service outcomes. Design the structure and process to address each part of professional practice: quality, competence, and practice.

Although there are four basic structures for shared governance and many adaptations of each, the councilor model (illustrated in Figure 2.7) is currently the most popular model used in practice at points of service in healthcare (Hess, 2009; Anthony, 2004; Porter-O'Grady, 1991, 2004; Swihart, 2011). Therefore, it will be presented here in greater detail for the purposes of developing the concepts and principles of shared governance implementation more fully.

Identifying competencies for engaging in shared governance, drawn from the conceptual model behind the most current instruments for measuring governance, is an important aspect of the design or redesign of shared governance. Competencies are written for:

- Design team members
- Leadership
- Point-of-service employees

Shared competencies for participating in councils, committees, and at points of service are embedded in the Index for Professional Nursing Governance (IPNG) and Index for Professional Governance (IPG), both of which can be found in the back of this book in Appendix A, as well as in your downloads (Appendixes 1 and 2, respectively). The tool in Appendix 5, the competency decision worksheet, and the council shared decision-making tool (see Appendix 4 for a sample worksheet, more information, and tips for decision-making) can help council members organize their information and reports of activities for sharing with other councils, committees, and task groups with a seven-step shared decision-making process. Shared decision-making is the *process* for shared governance through which individuals and teams identify and resolve problems and capitalize on opportunities. The seven-step shared decision-making process is:

Step 1. Identify opportunities and diagnose problems
Step 2. Identify objectives
Step 3. Generate alternatives
Step 4. Evaluate alternatives
Step 5. Reach decisions
Step 6. Choose implementation strategy
Step 7. Monitor and evaluate outcomes

Building competencies in processes associated with shared governance, including decision-making and others delineated in the IPNG and IPG tools, can help participants identify and build their competencies (see Appendix 6) for engaging in shared governance across the organization and progressing their activities for sharing with other councils, committees, and task groups.

NOTE: Keys for developing and verifying competencies
Be sure to include the following important qualities in your competency development program:
- *Listening*
- *Self-awareness*
- *Dealing with the pyramid (top-down)*
- *Foresight*
- *Coaching, not controlling*
- *Developing your colleagues*
- *Unleashing others' energy and intelligence*

Implementing a councilor model for shared decision-making

Here are the steps to take for implementing a councilor model:

1. **Design a framework** for discussing implementation of shared governance and setting the direction for reshaping and transforming professional practice.

2. **Evaluate the basic structure** of the selected model—in this case, the councilor model.

3. **Identify and simplify accountability** of disciplines. There are five basic constructs that can be separated or combined in the design structure of the central governing councils or bodies. All professional committees, task forces, and practice groups will eventually be folded into one or more of these disciplines and become part of a designated governing council (i.e., central council).

4. **Create a professional overlay** for designing individual elements of the structure. The accountabilities (practice, management, quality, education, and research) will be the basis of the formation of the governing councils, whether in five councils or some other designated grouping.

Establish a design team

The design team (i.e., steering group, coordinating group, redesign team) brings together members of the organization representing each key role in the system, including staff (majority members), interprofessional partners, multidisciplinary team members, management, and leadership to plan the activities of structural design and to prepare the systems, leadership, and staff to establish the emerging paradigm shifts necessary to implement and sustain shared governance. Begin by identifying the size, membership, purpose, and goals. Then, look carefully at the functions and tasks expected of the design team (shown in Figure 3.3) before moving on to roles and responsibilities.

1. **Design team size:** Limit size to about seven to 15 members. The larger the group, the less constructive it may be in finding consensus for making and implementing decisions.

2. **Design team membership:** The design team mix needs to represent the percentage distribution of the organization of management and direct-care staff (majority). Drawing from services

rather than practices or work units generally establishes a broader group but keeps the team small enough to be effective. Select interprofessional partners, service leaders, direct-care staff, and multidisciplinary team members so they form a partnership in designing, implementing, and communicating the process elements of shared governance from the beginning.

3. **Design team purpose:** Focus on designing the shared governance process structure that will evolve after implementation:
    - The entire design process falls under this group
    - This team coordinates all of the shared governance activities initially

4. **Design team goals:** The team is empowered to do the work:
    - *Plan shared governance.* Define and describe what shared governance is and what it will look like in this organization at the point of service for employees and service leaders. Identify the roles of the multidisciplinary team members, executive leadership, and internal and external stakeholders.
    - *Guide implementation.* Once the structure is designed and shared governance has been defined in terms of an implementation plan, the design team continues to guide the process. Over time, the design team may change names (e.g., coordinating council, service town hall, or service forum) and expand functions to facilitate the ongoing progress of shared governance.
    - *Help staff and leaders with transition.* Create a timetable for transition. Assess readiness. Complete predetermined activities and provide subsequent activities for group members once councils are established. Develop a mechanism for personal and professional transitioning, a way of acknowledging accomplishments, and a social or symbolic activity for the transition (Porter-O'Grady, 2004, 2009c).
    - *Evaluate progress.* Evaluate progress initially, at six months, then annually once shared governance is implemented: where you are, how far you have come, and what has to be done in light of the design or plan you set in motion. This is critical to measuring success (Hess, 1998a, 1998b).

Roles and responsibilities of the design team

The design team establishes the foundations for shared governance within the organization. Some of the many roles and responsibilities include the following:

1. *Learn about shared governance and how it works.* If the team members are responsible for designing the format for shared governance, they need as much knowledge as possible from the beginning stages through mature development and standardization of practice. Build an information base to understand and structure the work.

FIGURE 3.3	Shared governance steering group functions and tasks
Steering group (Design or redesign team)	• Service: Delivery service models; disciplines service design; roles; quality; process • Operations: Resources; linkage; planning; market strategy; implementation; compliance • Governance: Mission, strategy, priorities, policy, integration • Design and redesign: Structures, activities, implementation
Tasks	• Review existing organizational and service structures and how they interface with current care system design activities • Identify key elements of structural change needed to support process shifts at points of service (*i.e.*, macro, meso, and microsystems) • List structural supports needed to replace or strengthen care design at points of service within and across the organization • Develop a draft of the essential characteristics, responsibilities, and accountabilities of emerging roles in the new shared governance structure; include new roles in position descriptions or role charters • Sketch out the team, service pathways, and system council format for decision making across the healthcare system from points of service to policy and governance levels • Define and implement activities and change events needed to formally reshape the organizational structure • Set up education and development learning processes for changes in practice and collaboration, shifts in roles and responsibilities, performance expectations, service adjustments, and leadership outcomes associated with design of shared governance • Evaluate progress and adapt process as needed

SOURCES: Adapted from Edmonstone, J. (2003). *Shared Governance: Making It Work*. Chichester, West Susex, United Kingdom: Kingsham Press; and Porter-O'Grady, T. (2009c). *Interdisciplinary Shared Governance: Structuring for 21st Century Practice*. Sudbury, MA: Jones & Bartlett Publishers.

2. *Select a shared governance process structure or model.* Determine which shared governance structure or model applies to the organization based on its culture, goals, and strategic plan. The structure selected must be a good fit for the organization and for professional nursing practice. Expect this structure to be adapted initially and multiple times as it matures and conforms to the needs of the staff and the organization with more and more voices represented over time.

3. *Identify tasks and create a timeline.* Focus on what will occur at what time to evaluate elements of the process and ensure that everyone succeeds in finishing assigned tasks. Developing this process is a long-term event. It usually takes three to five years to fully implement

an effective, efficiently operating shared governance process model. Each stage of the process builds on previous stages. Evaluating each stage will be preliminary to beginning the next stage. The timeline becomes a guide to successfully implementing the process and to determining where you are along the way. It helps keep the destination visible so that all participants can move to accept and manage the many changes needed for shared governance (Black and Gregersen, 2008; Porter-O'Grady, 1991).

4. *Evaluate goals and process outcomes.* Emphasize goals and anticipated outcomes at the beginning of the process (e.g., higher levels of employee satisfaction, higher retention rates, and increased safety outcomes). Measure and evaluate goals intermittently along the way. Design or select tools for measuring progress in shared governance that allow for evaluation and adjustment in the process along the way as outcomes are achieved (see Appendix A to refer to the IPNG and IPG).

Designing governance councils

When establishing the selected shared governance process structure, identify how many councils (bodies or groups) will be established to include all five accountabilities or disciplines. Once the disciplines are accounted for, there is no right or wrong way to design the structure or process.

One organization elected to begin with five central governing councils: (1) management or leadership council, (2) practice council, (3) research and evidence-based practice council, (4) professional development and education council, and (5) quality council, in addition to the practice- or unit-level councils, which were connected to each of the other five councils. This allowed the service to slightly reduce the number of council meetings direct-care staff would need to attend while still maintaining representation in each central governing body. (In this book, a council is described separately for each accountability or discipline for further discussion.)

Begin by identifying the outcomes desired. Some organizations establish one council at a time to help employees transition more easily and successfully through the change process. Others establish the central governing councils and practice or unit councils together to promote interactivity, communication, and workflow. This book will address the councils and structures one at a time to better describe them in more detail and recommend an order of establishment for those organizations that choose that approach.

1. **Start with the management (or leadership) council.** Purpose and responsibilities are to provide guidance and linkage to the central governing councils and serve as a mechanism for the service executive, service leaders, and managers or supervisors to participate in activities related to the provision of care at points of service. The management or leadership council deals almost exclusively with resource issues and allocations. The role for service leaders and

managers or supervisors in shared governance is primarily servant-based, providing resources, support, opportunities, boundaries, and protection (i.e., from losing needed resources during annual budget allocations) for staff at points of service, thereby freeing staff to focus all of their experience, expertise, and education on caring for patients and improving service outcomes. The manager or supervisor:

- Appropriates necessary resources for the professionals in practice (human, fiscal, material, support, and systems)
- Centers service around the practicing professional at points of care
- Integrates (links) the shared governance process with the other services and roles
- Channels information to and from direct-care staff through practice- or unit-level councils to and from services and organizational leadership, when appropriate
- Identifies systems problems and generates necessary responses
- Communicates encouragement, support, and boundaries (e.g., tells direct-care staff when there is no budget for new equipment requested by the practice- or unit-level council, then helps them explore other options for getting the necessary resources)

Management frequently has the greatest amount of growth and change to undergo for shared governance to be successful. Empowered staff members assume new roles of responsibility, authority, equity, accountability, and ownership traditionally belonging to managers or supervisors, which can cause territorial, personality, and role conflicts during implementation of shared decisional processes. Service leaders will need educational programs to help them adapt to new behaviors, learn new roles, and develop new skills as their current role evolves from management to servant leadership, a much higher and more demanding form of leading. This will be a challenging process for them. Devoting time and resources to their transitional development in the transformation of their leadership roles is critical.

2. **Establish the practice- or unit-level councils.** This usually follows or correlates well with the implementation of the management or leadership council. Here is where it all comes together. Purpose and responsibilities are to promote autonomy, equity, partnership, shared accountability, and ownership for practice or unit operations by managing point-of-service care; measuring and documenting care outcomes (quality monitors and indicators); providing orientation, mentorships, and preceptorships for new employees, new graduates, the newly qualified, and students doing clinical rotations; participating in schedule development; sharing charge responsibilities; conflict management and problem solving; assessing and meeting educational needs and practice- or unit-specific competencies; engaging in evidence-based practice (research, journal clubs); monitoring practice- or unit-specific activities and safety

issues (policies, quality improvement, safety); and managing practice or unit education (in-services, mandatory training, continuing education).

3. **Develop a practice council.** Purpose and responsibilities are to set the criteria for evidence-based practice consistent with established and evolving professional standards and regulating agencies. This council keeps the development of the staff in concert with the changes of management and leadership roles. Most of the other councils' work will depend on the foundational work completed and managed by the practice council, which has the control and authority to make decisions affecting policies and practice for the work they do:
    - Defines, implements, and maintains practice
    - Selects theory base
    - Sets practice standards
    - Sets performance standards
    - Defines career advancement

4. **Initiate a quality council.** Purpose and responsibilities are to monitor and evaluate performance and outcome measurements based on evidence-based practice using the best scientific knowledge available, to provide a forum for multidisciplinary team collaboration, and to integrate quality initiatives into practice. The work of the quality council depends on the work of the management or leadership and practice councils. For example, the practice council's service standards need to be developed before the quality council can identify and develop measurement standards. Performance standards must be done before developing a performance evaluation system (quality council). Therefore, it is important to establish a deliberate, step-by-step relationship among the councils and a clear basis on which they can depend for their complementary development.

5. **The goal of shared governance** is that ownership and investment of all the workers and the outcome of the work ties back into how you define the work and how performance is measured against that definition. If the staff member defines the work, performs on that definition, and achieves work outcomes, he or she can also evaluate progress or individual performance related to that work. The quality council:
    - Monitors and measures standards of care. Establishing practice- or unit-level clinical quality council champions is one approach to interactive collaboration for continuous quality improvement. Appendix 7, sample commitment agreement for clinical quality champions, and Appendix 8, sample unit or clinical quality champion orientation, are tools used by the staff of the surgical ICU at St. Luke's Health System to establish such champions and orient them to their roles within practice- or unit-level councils and in partnership with the central governing quality council and the quality management systems.

- Designs the quality and performance improvement system and dashboards or scorecards.
- Controls the performance evaluation system (a peer-based process in shared governance, not management-based).
- Sets the goals for patient care monitoring (defines a standard of care, measures it, reaches it, and changes the standard so providers work at a higher level of function or outcome).
- Manages the credentialing and privileging program. Every professional provider has an obligation for the quality and type of work he or she does. Establishing a peer-based process for new employees when they first enter the organization that continues throughout their employment helps ensure a good fit with the organization and with discipline or service.

6. **Initiate a professional development and education council.** Purpose and responsibilities are to provide orientation; to assess ongoing learning and competency needs; and to define, implement, and maintain standards, continuing education, and in-services that promote professional and personal growth and ongoing competency of professional providers and their healthcare team members. The professional development and education council:

- Ensures professional competency in ongoing learning activities, the basis of performance measurement over the long term. This council facilitates implementation of competency mechanisms that ensure a continuous mechanism for education and development is present, is staff-based, and clearly represents the work done rather than some preplanned objective that may or may not reflect the practice- or unit-specific needs of the employees at points of service.
- Develops an effective communication network through each of the central and practice- or unit-level councils.
- Manages staff orientation programs and preceptorships, which are critical to the success of new employees (new graduates, managers or supervisors, agency and contract staff), and practice- or unit-specific or clinical orientations.
- Plans quarterly and annual staff meetings:
  » Quarterly meetings: Staff and council members get together to deal with issues of concern to the organization as a whole as it impacts disciplines and services; to report to the staff what activities they have been involved in; to get feedback from the staff about what is occurring; to relate, communicate, and interact; to look at goals and learning objectives for the year; to review activities and the progress of those activities over time; and to deal with operational issues.
  » Annual meetings: Staff and council members look at goals and objectives of the organization, discuss and report the annual learning needs assessment and education

plan, consider problems and issues of the discipline (education and professional development) as a whole, determine how to fit those issues with the goals of the organization, and review organizational problems and issues affecting the discipline. This is an opportunity to give awards for service and to acknowledge the contributions of those who have acted on behalf of the staff during the previous year. It can be an opportunity for formal and informal communication and celebration.

- Facilitates staff members' access to learning-teaching activities by bringing training to the practice or unit level. Balance, personal growth, and professional development are natural outcomes of shared governance activities. Facilitating practice- or unit-level education is a major goal of this council. The learning process, content, and activities become more real and meaningful when applied more directly to professional practice at the points of service.

7. **Establish a research and evidence-based practice council** (if applicable). This council follows the development of the previous two councils, quality and professional development. Not all organizations have well-defined research activities. However, one of the clinical accountabilities in shared governance is research. Professional providers need to be committed to validating old knowledge and discovering new knowledge, which is an integral part of the research process. Research seeks knowledge that will enhance patient care outcomes, offer a new basis for the work to be done at points of service, and help direct-care staff develop critical thinking skills, evidence-based practices, and abilities to understand and participate in research at points of service. This council is a way to formalize that process. It is often the last council implemented because it is the most dependent on the other councils being in place and is the most resource dependent.

8. **Create an advocacy council** (if applicable). This council is becoming more embedded in the culture of shared governance models and often works in concert with the professional development council. The advocacy council defines and maintains strategies that support all service employees. Members promote professional advancement, advocacy, and recognition through communication, coordination, and staff advocacy; recruitment and appreciation; and celebratory activities around practice, quality, and competency of healthcare providers at all levels. They work most closely with practice- or unit-level councils in identifying needs and developing their activities. Some of those activities include establishing and promoting relationships among all types of community organizations through contributions to practice and care outcomes and the health of the communities they serve (e.g., providing CPR training to the community during an annual CPR day). This council also seeks opportunities to acknowledge employees in various and substantive ways for their accomplishments, enhancing the image of healthcare providers in the organization and in the community, through awards ceremonies,

public announcements of certifications and promotions, and special events (e.g., collecting clothes and toiletries for the homeless). Because of the generally fun and celebratory atmosphere of this council, there are nearly always lots of volunteers to serve on it.

Focus on council membership

When recruiting members for the varied shared governance councils, there are a number of factors to consider: representation, contributions, membership mix, size of councils, length of time of participant service, and meeting times.

1. **Representation:** From a service context, these representatives will speak on behalf of those services when decisions have to be made.
2. **Contributions:** Contributions are made by each member over time; work may be assigned to members to be done in the meeting or taken back to their practices or units and completed there. Reports on tasks and progress are given at each council meeting.
3. **Membership mix:** Central governance councils (practice, quality, professional development, research) need to be composed of mostly direct-care staff, about 70% to 90% clinical staff. The other council members should be management or support staff. These are staff-driven councils. They will make staff decisions that affect clinical practice, quality, and competency. Messages of empowerment, equity, autonomy, and accountability are delivered in an effective and clear way so that shared decision-making emerges in partnership with the staff and management or leadership.
4. **Size of councils:** The number of participants depends on the number of disciplines, practices, or units represented. Usually, only seven to 15 members are recommended. However, there are organizations with more representatives at the table. It is important that all practices or units have someone at the table to represent their voices in the discussions and shared decision-making. The larger the groups, though, the more difficult it is to get consensus and make decisions. How to overcome this potential obstacle would have to be addressed by the design team when developing initial guidelines for the council structures and at the beginning of work in larger groups by the council members.
5. **Length of time of participant service:** It often takes about a year for a participant to learn the roles of assigned councils. Therefore, a two-year term seems to be emerging as the standard length of service commitment for each central governing council member. With a two-year term, consider rotating one-half of the members off one year and the other half off the second year. This rotation would provide continuity of process with at least half of the members having served for one year and able to orient and mentor the oncoming central council members. For practice- or unit-level councils, however, a one-year term seems to be the norm at present.

6. **Meeting times and structures:** How organizations elect to structure their council meetings and times will be dependent on factors unique to that staff:
    - Some councils meet once a month for eight hours (a full day) to accomplish the tasks of the council. This allows members to focus on the business of the council instead of dividing their attention or concern with the patients or tasks they left on the unit for an hour or two.
    - Other councils have a monthly "meeting day" when all councils meet, usually for an hour each, at different times to allow staff members to attend their meetings and return to work around the council meetings. Breaks of 15–30 minutes between council meetings allow staff members who serve on more than one central council to get to the next one without disrupting or interfering with the work of other councils.

- For example:
    - 8:00 a.m. to 9:00 a.m.: Management or leadership council
    - 9:30 a.m. to 10:30 a.m.: Quality council
    - 11:00 a.m. to 12:00 p.m.: Professional development and education council
    - 12:30 p.m. to 1:30 p.m.: Practice council
    - 2:00 p.m. to 3:00 p.m.: Research and evidence-based practice council (if one has been established)
    - 3:30 p.m. to 4:30 p.m.: Advancements, advocacy, and recognitions council (if one has been established)
- Council meetings cannot be optional. Attendance has to be mandatory if direct-care staff and service leadership are to have a voice in shared decision-making and be able to complete and communicate council activities. It is critical that service leadership support and facilitate staff attendance at assigned council meetings. It is also important to provide time and opportunity for communication of information and data gathering to complete council assignments (e.g., practice- or unit-level in-services). These are details to be discussed and resolved by each service leader, manager, or supervisor and his or her staff.

Each central council is structured with certain accountabilities or disciplines. Staff councils must have authorities identified that belong to the staff and operate within the practice framework. To be successful, the focus must be on empowered engagement of all participants.

Focus on shared governance empowerment process

Each central governing council selects a chair from among the membership to provide leadership for the council. For the staff councils, that chair will be selected from among the staff, the research council chair may be management or staff, and the management (or leadership) council selects its own chair. These chairs must be empowered to do the work of managing or leading the councils with the responsibility, authority, equity, ownership, and accountability to make decisions and to act on those decisions. Empowering the chair means the chair of each council will be given certain basic powers secured by the role. It is recommended that the chair will:

1. Be elected by peers
2. Control the agenda
3. Act for the group, speak for the group members, and make decisions for them when the group is not in session
4. Assign group tasks and functions
5. Move the group to decision-making when discussion indicates a need
6. Accept no additional assignments; this role is generally extensive and demanding enough without additional assignments
7. Remove nonperforming members from the group if necessary

Part 4. Bylaws and Articles

Formalizing the shared governance structure

You've got to think about "big things" while you're doing small things, so that all the small things go in the right direction.
—Alvin Toffler

During the formalization of the shared governance structures, the roles of management and implementation of shared decision-making are established in the clinical and work units of the organization. Principles that underpin shared governance are defined and their application to the organization as a whole are described. Activities following the beginning phases of implementation are completed. This process may take from three to five years to be fully established. At the end of that time, identify the activities that provide structure and context to the newly designed professional practice in ways that can be understood and replicated by participants in other parts of the organization.

Bylaws for shared governance process models

Developing and implementing bylaws are generally part of the formalization of the shared governance process (Porter-O'Grady, 1991, 2004). Bylaws may be either descriptive or prescriptive:

- *Prescriptive* bylaws set the rules on which an organization will evolve.
- *Descriptive* bylaws describe the organization already in place. Many groups prefer descriptive bylaws.

Organizational structure is established based on the design and implementation plan with each part of the structure in place. The bylaws, then, simply define the structure once the implementation process begins. When it occurs and is far enough along to give evidence of the operating structure that the participants want, look specifically at bylaws. (See Appendix 9, bylaws and guidelines for shared governance process models; Appendix 10, sample role descriptions for shared governance council members, chairs, cochairs, and secretaries; Appendix 11, sample set of central council bylaws; and Appendix 12, sample unit or practice council charter.)

When all the pieces come together, it is important to recognize that the work of the design team (steering group) ends at some point in the implementation process. By the end of the second or third year, the formative design stages of the organization end. It is important to transition to a more permanent council format to integrate the organizational system and operations before this occurs.

Emerging executive (operations or coordinating) council

The executive (operations or coordinating) council generally emerges from the context and operations of the transitioning design team, or steering group.

1. **Establish the council format:** Move from design team or steering committee to executive, operations, or coordinating council. Chairs of the individual councils are elected and nominated to assume leadership roles. Each of these elected chairs becomes a member of the executive council with the chief nurse executive or chief nurse officer of that particular service, division, or department.

2. **Council responsibility:** With the executive officer and the elected leaders of the councils, the executive (operations or coordinating) council takes form and becomes the decision-making body that integrates the organizational system and operations. It does not usurp or remove responsibilities or accountabilities from the central governing councils or from the practice- or unit-level councils. The executive (operations or coordinating) council is responsible for:

    - *Integration:* This is a fundamental responsibility of this group. In fact, the executive council has no accountability except the responsibilities designated to it by the central governing councils. It focuses on integration, conflict resolution, goal setting, operations, and bylaws.

    - *Conflict resolution:* Between and among central councils, between staff and councils, and between management and councils, the executive (operations or coordinating) council resolves conflict in the organization as a whole.

    - *Goal setting:* The council sets the goals and objectives for the division, reviews the budget, and settles those issues that are in question or need to be clarified to ensure that the set direction moves forward. It sees the structure and relationships in the organizational system operate effectively. The success of the system is dependent on the integration, coordination, and facilitation of its various functions.

- *Bylaws:* This group is responsible for the construction of the bylaws (see Appendix 9, bylaws and guidelines for shared governance process models; Appendix 10, sample role descriptions for shared governance council members, chairs, cochairs, and secretaries; and Appendix 11, a sample set of central council bylaws). They form, manage, control, adapt, and change the bylaws as needed. Change may come from anywhere in the organization. However, that change must be submitted to this elected and appointed executive, operations, or coordinating council to determine that it does not in some way harm the integrity of the organization. Afterwards, any changes recommended can be submitted to the executive council in a general session or at the annual meeting for inclusion in the bylaws revision and review. The bylaws then take form and can be adjusted legitimately and equitably without threatening the integrity of the organizational system. From this, leadership and direction for development of the governance process evolves.

3. **Leadership and governance:** Leadership emerges from all the places in the organizational system and operations. Direct-care staff leadership is essential to the successful implementation of shared governance. The leadership role of the manager or supervisor, too, is critical. This role changes dramatically in the terms of behavior modification, development, and exercising the management role as shared governance processes create new behaviors essential to success in the new structural process model.

Importance of the manager or supervisor

The manager or supervisor is the gatekeeper and key to the success of shared governance implementation. These individuals guide the developmental processes and must adapt to new, broader characteristics of their roles as they support those processes.

1. Developmental processes occur at different rates in different places but with the same outcomes. Empowered organizations cannot be managed in the same way as traditional organizations. As direct-care staff mature in their professional behaviors and exercise ownership and accountability, those new behaviors will impact the role of the manager or supervisor. Clearly, managers and supervisors in the organizational system and operations are needed—it is a myth to assume that the management process disappears in empowerment processes. The role evolves into exemplified, servant leadership due to the resource nature of the role.

2. New characteristics of the role are broader. In the traditional definition of the role, the manager or supervisor was the planner, leader, organizer, and controller of the system. The empowering manager or supervisor will develop other characteristics (coordinator, facilitator, integrator), with the ability to pull those pieces together and to exemplify those roles in a shared decision-making model. This is critical to the manager or supervisor's success in

applying the new role and exercising it to make a difference in the resources available for the direct-care staff decision-makers.

Practice- or unit-level councils in shared governance

In the midst of the shared governance process, the practice- and unit-level councils must be well established (see Appendix 12, unit and practice council charter, and Appendix 13, shared governance central council charter). Shared governance cannot make a difference if the practices or units do not establish their own councils representing their own culture and designed in a way that fulfills their own needs and concerns in the central governing councils. The only caveat for this process is that the practices and units fulfill the principles directed for them by the central governance councils and provided for them in the organizational structure and operations. Using these principles and applying them to the practice and unit councils will ensure there will be organizational consistency and the organization as a whole will implement shared governance successfully.

In the final analysis, it is important to know shared governance is not the property of any individual, department, division, or discipline. It is a universal organizational management process model, a way of working together to accomplish goals and objectives that invests all the participants in shared decision-making, partnership, equity, accountability, and ownership. It is a practical approach for reshaping and transforming professional practice at points of service.

Redesigning Shared Governance

Life can only be understood looking backward,
but can only be lived looking forward.
    —*Søren Kierkegaard*

Establishing the infrastructure, councils, and linkages necessary to create a successful implementation of shared governance process is difficult and complex. All transformation requires significant investment of time, commitment, and resources. Shared governance is not management by committee, council, or leadership. It is an accountability-based approach to decision-making and shared leadership. Roles of managers and supervisors must mature significantly to those of coach, mentor, preceptor, advisor, and resource manager. The demands and complexities of the organization, management, and the staff inherent in such a transition can occasionally stall the process.

A breakdown in the implementation process can occur for many reasons. The organization may then decide to:

- Stop implementing shared governance and reinstate the old paradigms;
- Proceed with the original design once the problems are identified and addressed, advancing the work begun by the first steering group; or,

- Reassess the situation, select a steering group to redesign the structures and processes for beginning again, and for advancing the implementation of shared governance.

Once a decision has been made to redesign the shared governance structures and processes, it is important to bring the stakeholders together. Provide a format for the work to be done, allowing for adaptation and change, fostering relationships and systems linkages, and rebuilding support systems with all the elements needed to make the system successful and sustainable going forward. Redesigning the structures and processes can lead to a stronger, more resilient shared governance management process going forward.

Chapter 4

Building the Practice and Unit Councils

*Never tell people how to do things.
Tell them what to do and they
will surprise you with their ingenuity.*
—George S. Patton

Why Are Practice and Unit Councils So Important?

The practice or unit council is the core structure for shared governance in healthcare. Practice and unit shared governance provides a critical forum to give all direct-care providers assigned to a particular practice or unit an opportunity to participate in shared decisional processes and outcomes specific to the needs and activities of that practice or unit. Although all staff of all levels may participate, practice and unit councils are led and managed by the direct-care provider. Members of practice and unit councils identify, explore, and resolve issues, questions, ideas, and concerns related to professional practice, quality, competency, education, and the work environment. But first, they must ask themselves some difficult questions, such as:

- What is my role in shared governance?
- How do I view the practice environment, leadership, interprofessional partnerships, multidisciplinary teams, professional practice model, and patient-care delivery systems?
- What do I want to contribute at the practice or unit level? At the department or division level? At the organization level? At the community level?
- What support is available for the additional time needed to participate equitably in shared governance at the varied levels of responsibility and accountability?

- What resources and skills do I need to be successful in my professional role on this unit or in this practice? In this organization?

Once they have explored their own possible contributions and ideas about shared governance, members of the practice or unit council should challenge themselves with the following questions as they move forward to help build and expand the practice or unit council:

1. Are we doing it right?
    - Are direct-care staff members leading the practice or unit council?
    - Is the manager or supervisor supportive of staff participating in the practice or unit council and related and assigned activities?
    - Are human, material, and fiscal resources (e.g., time, staffing, and supplies) available for the work of the practice or unit council?
    - Is provider participation in the practice or unit council by invitation or mandated?
    - Is there a formal structure for holding meetings and reporting outcomes?

2. Are we doing the right thing well?
    - Are managers, providers, and staff appropriately involved in the practice or unit council when needed?
    - Is the agenda appropriate and manageable for the time allocated for the practice or unit council meeting?
    - Is there a facilitator to help participants achieve the desired outcomes and the meeting objectives?
    - Is the practice or unit meeting coordinated well enough to ensure continuity and participation by members while others manage patient care?
    - Are meetings and activities (i.e., quality dashboards, safety, contributions to practice policies, evidence-based practice, point-of-care research) managed in an efficient manner with due consideration given to allocation of resources to engage in shared decision-making and shared leadership at point of service and to address issues related to practice, quality, and competence?

3. Do job descriptions and functional statements for providers reflect the language of shared governance related to professional practice, autonomy, ownership, equity, partnership, responsibility and accountability, authority, quality, and competency?

Dealing With Change

Building the practice or unit council for implementing shared governance at points of service is about change—how do we make change painless?

> *Change has a considerable psychological impact on the human mind.*
> *To the fearful it is threatening because it means that things may get worse.*
> *To the hopeful it is encouraging because things may get better.*
> *To the confident it is inspiring because the challenge exists to make things better.*
> —King Whitney, Jr.

With changing technology, increasing acuities, patients and families who are more knowledgeable about healthcare, and emerging paradigm shifts, change is our only constant. Healthcare providers must embrace new skills, take more professional risks, and reach further than ever before. What an exciting time.

Yet nobody actually likes change. New technologies and processes, skills, and professional demands seem costly, risky, frighteningly complicated, and too time-consuming to learn. The resulting stress can make providers feel increasingly overwhelmed and overworked. Change occurs so quickly that unfreezing from past behaviors is no longer possible before new demands consume our attention. There is rarely time to become comfortable with new information before it is being replaced with even newer ideas, processes, and concepts with a promise of higher quality and lower cost. The answer: partnerships and strategies to help providers accept change and realize future possibilities.

Change may not be an option, but how to engage in it is open to negotiation and does not have to be painful (Schoemer, 2009):

- Begin with the right attitude
- Let your confidence show
- Be autonomous in practice and presence
- Be an expert learner
- Be solution-oriented
- Speak up
- Create and innovate

- Let integrity rule
- Communicate and relate
- Strike a balance between work and play
- Become a teacher, preceptor, coach, mentor
- Be a student of the business of healthcare
- Be adaptive
- Be a transformational (servant) leader, formally and informally

Transformational (Servant) Leadership

Healthcare providers understand and practice transformational (or servant) leadership at every level of care—it begins with a desire to serve others. Such service has the power to transform the lives of those who serve and those who are served. It builds relationships with meaning, purpose, and respect. It is unique to the one who has the ability to serve and lead. Power is not coercive. It is used to create opportunity and alternatives so that others may choose and build autonomy.

Transactional leaders (those who use a power model of leadership, sometimes referred to as *command-and-control leaders*) are more evident in most healthcare organizations at all levels. They are not problematic to the success of an organization and are often good, intelligent, vital people who manage tasks, events, programs, resources, and technology quite well. Problems arise when they try to manage rather than lead people. Frequently, positional power or authority is used to coerce, intimidate, or control staff rather than engage them. The relationship frequently has a parental feel to it.

Transforming leaders (sometimes referred to as *influencing,* or *servant leaders*) are more complex and potent than other leaders. This leader recognizes an existing need or demand and then looks beyond it to motive and greater need (i.e., Maslow's hierarchy), and engages the whole person. The result is an adult-to-adult relationship of mutual trust, inspiration, respect, and potential that elevates staff members to servant leaders. Such leaders are transformative.

A *transforming leader,* then, is simply a leader intent on serving others, one who loves people and wants to help them. Because transformational leadership is first and foremost an act of service, it transforms two internal and two external domains of the one who would lead:

- Internal
    » Heart—motivations: self-serving (egocentric) vs. serving others
    » Head—leadership point of view
- External
    » Hands—public leadership behaviors
    » Habits—habits as by others

Leadership is about moving from a self-serving heart to a serving one. True leadership is about what we give, rather than what we get (Blanchard and Hodges, 2003; Greenleaf, 1991, 2008; Nightingale, 1858, 1992).

When healthcare providers approach shared governance with the same genuineness they employ in patient care, they will find these transformative qualities in their own leadership and expressed in the collaborative relationships they build. A practice or unit council is not another work group. It is a unique structure for providers to practice their profession through shared decisional processes and transformational, servant leadership.

Building Relationships

Interprofessional and multidisciplinary teams

Healthcare providers do not work in silos. Healthcare organizations are incredibly complex macrosystems. Although practice and unit councils operate at the microsystem level, it is important for direct-care providers and staff working at points of service to think about the big picture when building relationships.

The pharmacy staff at one facility were becoming overwhelmed with the growing number of demands and stat orders from a particular medical-surgical nursing unit. Some nurses were adding "stat" to requests to expedite their orders rather than because of actual need. After several attempts to speak to the behaviors and explain the escalating problems they caused in the pharmacy, the chief of pharmacy services asked to attend a unit council meeting. He never mentioned the tension among staff members or how busy his own team was, though. Instead, during the council meeting, he invited the nurses to tour the pharmacy after lunch and arranged for them to see their new technology and services.

They did—and arrived at the busiest, most chaotic time of the day. Machines shouted. Orders flew. Telephones shrieked. Patients demanded. The pharmacy staff took it all with grace (mostly), dignity, and a herculean effort to respond to every request, shout, shriek, and demand. The nurses watched in awe and left with greater respect for the pharmacy staff's workload. Thanking the chief, the nurses returned to their units, scheduled a special council meeting with a representative from the pharmacy to participate in their discussion, and tackled the problem. Together, they collaborated on new guidelines for how the nurses could manage pharmacy orders more efficiently and what pharmacy staff could contribute equitably. The relationships they built continue to thrive and grow.

The practice or unit council offers an opportunity for providers to take control of their own practice; to engage with interdisciplinary team members, interprofessional partners, leadership, patients and families, and guests from other communities of practice and points of service; and to build the relationships essential to successful patient-care outcomes. When selecting tools, setting up a practice or unit council, and determining what to add to the agenda, providers include important linkages with:

- Interprofessional partners and other multidisciplinary team members (e.g., physicians, nurses, pharmacists, managers or supervisors, clinical nurse leaders, dietitians, pharmacy representatives, advanced practice nurses, educators and staff development specialists, social workers, chaplains, environmental services)

- Central governance councils
- Organization and service line committees and task or work groups
- Communities of practice (i.e., those who share a profession and engage in a process of collective learning through interaction and shared decision-making)
- Communities of service and engagement with and service to members of local communities (i.e., a practice council that provides CPR training to local schools as a community or public service each year)

With continuous change inherent in the work we do, keeping pace with those changes and making appropriate adjustments in our approach to engaging in shared governance are a constant challenge. Recognizing this, we would like to take a fresh look at practice and unit councils here and offer some sample tools and techniques to help guide implementation and improvements in establishing a strong structure and shared decisional processes.

The tools and templates included in this book and on its download Web page were developed and selected in response to requests received over the past five years from healthcare providers engaged in shared governance, at both the practice and unit level. Choose those that best fit your purposes and adapt them to add value and reduce the amount of time and effort required to establish and advance your councils.

NOTE: *See the list of figures and tools page for a complete cataloging of sample tools included on the download Web page. At the end the book, you'll also find an extensive bibliography that presents additional readings and research on shared governance.*

Building the Structure for Practice and Unit Councils

Step 1: Create your design team or steering committee
Select a structure for designing and steering development of a model for unit councils.

Consider the following activities:
1. **Establish a design team or steering committee of staff members** to develop the structures and guiding principles for practice and unit councils. Because this structure is provider-driven, the majority of team members should be direct-care staff with input from managers or supervisors and the executives. This team develops the initial model and infrastructure of practice and unit councils and provides tools to help employees implement the templates at points of service. Practice and unit teams will then further develop their councils according to their own work and goals.

2. **Select a chair for the design team.** If this person is a direct-care employee, a cochair might be a manager to provide guidance, resources, and boundaries as work evolves.

3. **Select a liaison or facilitator for the design team.** This person facilitates communication within the department or service, among the staff as the practice or unit councils are being formed, and as a contact person for the governing councils and service leaders. Although not required, a liaison or facilitator helps free up the other members of the design team or steering committee to do the work of developing the practice or unit council structures, processes, and targeted outcomes. Once the practice and unit councils are established, a facilitator can continue to monitor and oversee long-term practice and unit projects.

4. **List the key drivers for practice and unit councils** (e.g., professional practice, quality and safety, competency and professional excellence, evidence-based practice and research, peer review, best practices, collaborative relationships, awards and recognition, operations), as distinguished from accountabilities for shared decision-making and collaborations of service leaders and direct-care staff (Haag-Heitman and George, 2010; Porter-O'Grady, 2009a, 2009b, 2009c), including:

   - Service leaders (i.e., managers and supervisors):
     » Administrative operations and resources (human, material, fiscal)
     » Work environment and structure to facilitate autonomy and professionalism
     » Organization (macrosystem) and department (mesosystem) linkages
     » Rewards and recognitions related to performance appraisals and evaluations
     » Strategic planning

   - Direct-care providers:
     » Practice and unit councils and practice operations
     » Standards of practice (specialty and clinical competencies; professional practice models)
     » Care delivery systems
     » Professional development (clinical and academic activities; orientation, preceptorships, and mentorships; continuing education and certifications)
     » Quality improvement (evidence based practice, research, quality outcomes)
     » Peer review (competency, performance evaluations, 360-degree assessments, feedback)
     » Multidisciplinary team relationships and interprofessional partnerships
     » Service-specific strategic planning

Step 2: Develop the formal framework and bylaws
Develop the unit council bylaws or charter.

Discuss key drivers identified and select a framework for the operations and management of the practice or unit council, usually bylaws or a charter (see Appendix 12 for a sample unit or practice charter). Simple guiding principles generally are not strong enough to establish the practice or unit council as a formal structure for shared governance. Bylaws and charters, documents describing the formal organization and operations of the practice or unit council and membership, emphasize the importance of the councils and their professional activities.

1. Develop a generic set of practice or unit council bylaws or a charter with formal descriptions for all levels of participation, responsibilities, and accountabilities:
   - Membership (nominations, term limits, commitment, dismissal from service)
   - Meetings and timelines (how often and for how long; set calendar for at least a year at a time)
2. Describe how communications (respectful, open, honest, focused) will:
   - Be disseminated among staff on all shifts and off-tours (e.g., weekends and holidays)
   - Flow within and among units and other practice settings (e.g., email, bulletin boards, SharePoint sites, newsletters, staff meetings)
   - Flow between and among governing (central) councils (see Appendix 13, sample shared governance council consult form; Appendix 14, sample communication policy; Appendix 15, sample communication flow chart; Appendix 16, sample council attendance form; and Appendix 17, sample council agenda and minutes)
3. Responsibilities and accountabilities:
   - Direct-care staff
   - Service leadership
   - Clinical nurse leaders (quality systems and performance measures)
   - Clinical educators and staff development specialists
   - Advanced practice nurses and physician assistants, for example
   - Interprofessional and multidisciplinary team members (when invited to a meeting)

Step 3: Make council meetings productive
Determine what happens in a unit practice council meeting.

People frequently complain about time spent in meetings and may consider them largely a waste of time and resources. However, meetings are critical to advancing shared governance, regardless of what form they take. In meetings, important discussions and key decisions are purposefully made that shape processes and determine actions. It is frequently in the context of meetings that teams are formed, tested, and strengthened, for example, by:

- Exchanging and evaluating information, consults, research, processes, actions
- Problem solving and conflict management
- Exploring opportunities for continual improvement and shared decision-making

In spite of this, many people struggle with finding a format that facilitates the positive outcomes possible with an engaged team and creating a structure, purpose, and process for participating in meaningful meetings. What are some of the challenges that can stall progress? What happens in council meetings to facilitate effective, efficient, and productive meetings?

Challenges can begin when *consensus* becomes *compromise* and collective decisions become:

- *Analysis paralysis*: Time and progress are lost as excessive details are explored, questioned, discussed, and argued so much other objectives may not be addressed.
- *Legacy thinking:* We've always done it that way. If it's not broken, why fix it? This is just the latest flavor of the month—why bother changing anything now?
- *Groupthink:* The group begins to collectively think as with one mind with uncritical acceptance or conformity to a particular point of view, more concerned with maintaining unity than with objectively evaluating their situation, to reason or discuss alternative actions or ideas and options.

To get the most out of council meetings, begin by remembering every meeting is unique, with its own purpose, objectives, agenda, and expected outcomes. Its success is determined by the actions, changes, progress, and improvements resulting from the meeting. Always remember meetings are about active engagement of all attendees. While the chair and cochair bear primary responsibility for conducting council meetings, each attendee has his or her own responsibilities and accountabilities for managing and evaluating them—for example, the secretary, recorder, facilitator, member, advisors, and guests all have specific roles and contributions to ensure the successful council meeting outcomes.

Build your shared governance council toolkit

The following tools and ideas can help you build a toolkit to facilitate productive, creative, and transformative decisions to advance shared governance through shared governance council meetings.

1. Start with an agenda and minutes (see Appendix 18, sample unit or practice council agenda and minutes template; Appendix 19, sample unit or practice council minutes with notes; and Appendix 20, sample council sign-in form).

2. Topics for discussion and decision-making (related to practice, quality, and competence) include:

- Clinical practice (grounded in evidence-based practice and practice-based evidence)
- Participatory and self-scheduling
- Time management (i.e., organization, prioritization, and delegation)
- Quality management systems and performance measures (i.e., the plan-do-check-act process)
- Professional development and education (see Appendix 21, a guideline for performance improvement in shared governance)
- Peer review (professional and institutional, performance, and competency; see Appendix 22, sample peer evaluation form)
- Research and evidence-based practice at points of service
- Journal club (see Appendix 23 for articles, action plans, and after-action reviews; see Appendix 24 for a guide to journal clubs)
- Service or department administration and leadership (role of manager or supervisor in practice or unit council meetings)
- Financial stewardship at points of service and improved fiscal outcomes
- Contributing to strategic plans (see Appendix 25, strategic planning with SWOT analysis template; Appendix 26, sample strategic planning tool; and Appendix 27, sample council strategic planning tool)
- Sample tools to help unit and practice councils with discussion and decision-making include:
  » Unit or practice council worksheet (see Appendix 28) to help identify specific topics related to categories of shared leadership and shared decisional opportunities
  » Council ground rules (see Appendix 29) to establish the basic expectations and structure for council meetings
  » Council discussion planner (see Appendix 30) to help focus discussions for projects, expectations, decisions, actions, reporting of outcomes, and follow-up related to topics and events under discussion
  » Council shared decision-making tool (see Appendix 4) to guide processes for shared decision-making within the shared governance structures and build more effective teams

Map out your council meeting

Putting it all together: What might a council meeting look like? The greatest part of an effective meeting is preparation, which happens before the meeting ever takes place:

- Identify purpose and objectives of the meeting
- Follow up on actions assigned during previous meeting
- Collect data or information requested to meet one or more objectives
- Prepare reports for agenda (e.g., may be asked to submit to secretary for inclusion with agenda prior to meeting so attendees can discuss the points of the report before or during the meeting—any council consults submitted or requiring follow-up since previous meeting)
- Invite subject matter or practice experts to attend meetings as appropriate to address questions or requests for more information (e.g., questions from a previous meeting) or those who can speak to agenda items from upcoming meeting
- Prepare the agenda and disperse to attendees; include minutes from previous meeting if they have not already been distributed
- Collect any comments, ideas, concerns, or other requests from attendees to be added to the agenda (e.g., under *New Business*)

Once the preparations have been completed, it is time to meet. The following example explores the flow of a council meeting with some tools to facilitate completing objectives and identifying actions to advance the work and opportunities of shared governance:

- Welcome attendees and make introductions (especially of guests)—make sure everyone has signed in (see Appendix 20, sample council sign-in form)
- Establish ground rules, which may be informal or formal; formal ground rules may address some of the same targets as council bylaws, e.g., council membership, attendance and participation, workload, reporting relationships and consults, resources, and amendments (see Appendix 29, sample unit or practice council ground rules)
- Review minutes from previous council meeting and approve, disapprove (e.g., for corrections or clarification of recorded notes), or approve with corrections
- Manager or supervisor's visit (usually 5–10 minutes) for information sharing or to receive requests or comments from council members, to provide encouragement, and to support the work of the council
- Presentations and discussions by guests, if present (e.g., infection control nurse, representative from a central council requested to bring more information or guidance or address council consults from staff, dietitian, researcher)
- Address new business (e.g., topic identified and discussed, responsibilities and assignments given, target dates and deadlines set)

- Address old business (e.g., previous topics and assignments discussed, follow-up, target dates and deadlines met)
- Recommendations for next agenda
- Adjournment
- Report of meeting minutes completed and disseminated to manager, supervisors, and all staff:
    » After-action reviews and activities (e.g., changing practice, building competency, preceptoring and mentoring, advancing improvements in quality, safety, and efficiency; see Appendix 23, sample after action review form, and Appendix 31, sample council quarterly report form)
    » Celebrations (celebrating coworkers and team members, such as graduations, certifications, ideas, promotions and advancements, accomplishments, best practices, birthdays, and anniversaries)

Meetings provide a forum for achieving genuine consensus and create opportunities for shared decision-making and leadership, and for engaging in shared governance across the organization to impact positive change and progress. Chairs, cochairs, secretaries, and facilitators often carry the greater responsibility for managing council meetings. Tips for managing meetings shared by others who do so can help them become more confident and comfortable in their roles.

Step 4: Plan for change

Explore ways to change practice and influence organizational outcomes through strategic planning and actions.

Shared governance, especially when first implemented, is a major change in an organization. Therefore, employees need to orchestrate the change in the most meaningful way possible for all members actively and passively engaged in the process. All practice levels of staff participate in developing the service strategic plan, the key to a successful implementation. They develop an organizing framework, a measurement tool, timeline, and list of accountabilities assigned to each of the central governance councils and the practice and unit councils (see Appendix 26, sample strategic planning tool). The service, discipline, or department executive provides the organizational strategic plan to ensure alignment of the service and practice or unit plans with the organization's overarching mission, vision, key drivers, and strategic goals (Haag-Heitman and George, 2010).

Strategic planning begins at the practice or unit level and involves all levels of employees in the process. Your strategic plan is a road map for ensuring that leadership and staff members are aligned and going in the right direction. As you create the plan, you will go through a process for identifying strategies and making decisions on allocating practice and unit resources to achieve specific outcomes around practice, quality, and competency.

*The difference between where we are
and where we want to be is what we do.*
—Author Unknown

Strategic planning helps leadership and staff members determine where a unit (department and organization) is going over the next year or longer, usually three to five years. To do this, the practice or unit council needs to know exactly where it is currently, then decide where it wants to go and how it will get there. Begin by conducting an *environmental scan,* a process for collecting data to answer questions about the present and future of the practice or unit, department, and organization using such tools as surveys, questionnaires, focus groups, and open forums to:

- Develop a common perception
- Identify strengths, weaknesses, trends, and conditions
- Draw on internal and external information

Strategic planning produces ideas and actions. Various techniques can be used in strategic planning, including *SWOT analysis,* a systematic look at strengths, weaknesses, opportunities, and threats developed by Albert Humphrey at Stanford Research Institute in the 1960s. SWOT analysis is useful in decision-making for multiple situations and activities, for identifying ideas and seeing how they relate to each other (see Appendix 25, sample strategic planning with SWOT analysis template). These headings provide a good framework for reviewing strategy, position, ideas, and direction of a practice or unit council. It also works well in brainstorming meetings and team-building exercises. (For more information and many free tools for implementing this approach to problem solving and strategic planning, check out the SWOT analysis method and examples, with a free SWOT template at *www.businessballs.com.*)

In strategic planning, you may:

- Describe the situation and set goals, objectives, and outcomes
- Conduct a SWOT analysis based on the identified goals
- Establish actions and processes needed to achieve these goals
- Implement agreed-upon actions, processes, changes in practice, etc., to operationalize the plan
- Monitor and get feedback from responsible person(s)
- Recognize benchmarks and deadlines when met
- Communicate changes made in practice, improvements in safety and patient care, and other achievements related to outcomes of strategic planning
- Evaluate and update strategic plans; identify methods for periodic review, evaluation, and revision to ensure plans and actions are aligned and on track

The primary purpose for strategic plans is *action*—translating strategies into day-to-day projects and the tasks required to achieve the plan. One way to keep individual workloads at a manageable level is to delegate different topics to *ad hoc* teams (e.g., a journal club, a quality improvement team, and a policies and procedures work group). The goals of practice or unit strategic planning must fit with the department or division and organizational strategic plans.

When involved in strategic planning, consider these important questions regarding governance and equity:

1. Strategic planning around *governance*:
   a. What existing policies, procedures, and statutes encourage or inhibit the strategic planning at the practice or unit level?
   b. How will the introduction of strategic planning affect the way the practice or unit works?
   c. How will the practice or unit council participants adjust to make the best use of strategic planning and implementation?
   d. How can the strategic plan be used to improve all aspects of the practice or unit council's operation?
   e. How will staff and leadership know if the strategic plan's objectives have been met?
   f. How will decisions about resources, schedules, practice, competencies, and patient safety and care be made?
   g. Will these decisions be part of the larger strategic plans for the department or division and organization?

2. Strategic planning around *equity*:
   a. How can strategic planning and implementation of changes benefit all staff?
   b. How will staff on all shifts and those unable to participate in strategic planning benefit from the changes?
   c. How can strategic planning benefit direct-care employees?
   d. How can strategic planning benefit resistant or disengaged staff, or those who are not performing well?

As you develop key strategies, analyze the practice or unit and its environment as it currently exists and envision how it may develop in the future. The final SWOT analysis helps staff identify multiple ideas, questions, and issues, and agree on those ideas relatively quickly. Your outcomes form the consensus on themes or ideas generated by the practice or unit council, department, or organization.

This is best achieved when employees:
- Participate in practice or unit council strategic planning
- Participate in service-level (department or division) strategic planning
- Participate in organization-level strategic planning

The analysis has to be executed at an internal level as well as an external level to identify all opportunities and threats of the external environment as well as the strengths and weaknesses of the practice or unit, the department, and the organization.Once the strategic plan is in place, it must be communicated.

Collaborate and communicate with all stakeholder groups. Engage all practice or unit staff and interprofessional and multidisciplinary team members in the strategic plan and outcomes. When others are engaged, they have an opportunity to participate and provide input.

Step 5: Facing challenges and troubleshooting
Troubleshoot obstacles and meet challenges to shared governance at points of service.

When we are no longer able to change a situation,
we are challenged to change ourselves.
    —Victor Frankl

Meeting challenges at points of service (i.e., engagement, disengagement, resistance):
- **Petulant participants** (Hess, n.d.). Managers and supervisors communicate to all staff that shared governance and the activities in the practice or unit council are not optional. Even then, some people will resist. It is important to engage them to:
    » Pull everyone in through education about what shared governance is and what it can do for their practice; emphasize the importance the organization ascribes to the shared governance program and activities; eliminate nonparticipation as an option
    » Assess and develop direct-care employees' knowledge and experience in leading and participating in shared decisional processes; staff may have been managed (often micromanaged) for so long they withdraw, having become comfortable with tasked assignments, and may fear the added responsibility and accountability inherent in shared governance; provide education, mentoring, and opportunities for them to participate fully in shared governance
    » Organize an involvement-friendly environment that is as easy as possible for all staff who are interested in doing so to attend meetings; shift focus from the individual to

the group; praise the enthusiasm of participants; build a sense of commitment and ownership

» Shared governance is not appropriate for every healthcare organization and not right for every provider; true detractors can make one of three choices:

- Refuse to participate and accept decisions from the group
- Participate informally in limited activities without attending formal meetings
- Refuse to participate on any level and, eventually, move on to find a better fit elsewhere

» Make sure everyone has the job- and role-appropriate skills needed for shared governance; do not confuse expertise with position or role

» Set a realistic time frame for achieving goals; give staff time, information, and encouragement—not everyone joins in at the same rate or time; as changes are made, benchmark and chart progress

- **Troublesome managers or supervisors.** These are often individuals placed in positions of leadership without sufficient orientation or training to prepare them for their roles, especially in areas of shared governance, transformational leadership, crucial conversations, and managing workplace complexities:

  » Many managers and supervisors are experienced in transactional leadership, often grounded in how they were managed early in their own careers and what they draw on when placed in leadership roles. Provide education and mentoring in transformational leadership skills.

  » Frequently, individuals were promoted into management or supervisory positions and service leader roles because of their clinical expertise, not their skills in either management or leadership. Educate, mentor, and encourage them in building knowledge, skill, and confidence.

  » Shared governance may elicit fear (i.e., **f**alse **e**vidence **a**ppearing **r**eal) in managers and supervisors asked to delegate tasks to staff they had always considered "their" job. Engage them in new roles, facilitate letting go of legacy systems, and help them develop new skills.

  » Some managers and supervisors refuse to adapt and engage in shared governance—they will not support their staff in transitioning into autonomous professional practice or align themselves with the direction of the organization in implementing shared governance. In such cases, the service executive may set a realistic time frame and participation goals for these managers and supervisors to achieve. They do not have the same gift of time as staff to engage. As leaders, they must be among the first on board with shared governance or it will not occur at points of service or organizationally.

» Shared governance needs to be built into the service strategic plan with supporting education, resources, and accountabilities for managers and supervisors, who are critical to the success of shared governance. They:

- Establish a work environment to support shared governance

- Set expectations of staff participation in practice and unit councils, committees, and central councils

- Facilitate staff readiness to change, adapt, and evaluate their own practice, quality, and competency, and to engage in participatory scheduling and peer reviews

- Manage staffing patterns and resources to support staff involvement in practice or unit council

- **Hesitant participants.** Find the underlying cause that holds them back and address it. The following examples of concerns by many direct-care providers about engaging in shared governance activities were taken from multiple employee satisfaction surveys and have been reported in the literature since the first edition of this book was published:

    » Too much responsibility and accountability but not enough authority

    » Not enough control over schedules

    » A perceived gap (communication and interaction) between administration and service, discipline, or profession

    » Manager or supervisor does not support shared governance or practice and unit councils

    » Not enough opportunities for advancement or education

    » Lack of autonomy

    » Lack of respect and collegiality from interprofessional partners

    » Not enough opportunity for staff to participate in administrative decision-making processes

    » Little or no voice in the planning of practice or unit policies and procedures, determining competencies, or managing their own performance measures and outcomes

- » Little or no time or resources given to participate in decision-making processes
- » Service administrators do not consult with staff on daily problems or procedures at points of service

- **Isolated practice or unit councils.** Make sure the structures and lines of communication are established before or during the establishment of practice and unit councils. Some organizations will set up a pilot council to see how it functions prior to developing the entire shared governance infrastructure. Although this approach may have some success, it can cause an imbalance or disconnect between the earlier established council and those that follow (i.e., when a microsystem becomes self-sufficient and autonomous without interacting with other central, practice, or unit councils, interprofessional and multidisciplinary teams, and external stakeholders, it can lead to isolation and an inability to fit readily back into the whole of the organization's shared governance macrosystem or service mesosystems).

- **Scheduling challenges.** The needs of direct-care providers and staff to provide safe, quality patient care always takes precedence, but implementing a shared governance program does require dedicated time.
  - » To facilitate time for regularly scheduled practice or unit council meetings in the face of patient-care priorities, meetings may need to be shortened or held by email, for example, to continue the operations of the practice or unit council.
  - » Direct-care providers need time away from the practice or unit and patient-care assignments to work on projects and assignments for the practice or unit council (or a committee or central council) to help advance practice at points of service, do research, or improve staff competencies. Managers and supervisors are critical in helping employees do the important work of the practice or unit council and still meet the patient-care needs of often exceedingly busy units.

- **Buy-in from the other staff and direct-care providers.** Many direct-care providers have only a vague idea of what council or committee members do at meetings or during time away from the practice or unit. To gain buy-in, do the following:
  - » *Communicate.* This is key: Share minutes and information about projects with staff. Invite them to contribute their own thoughts and talents to completing assignments.
  - » Negotiate schedules to allow equitable time for everyone to have special consideration of their requests whenever possible.
  - » Adjust staffing during governance meetings. One organization hired resource nurses to cover unit patient-care assignments while regular staff participated in their shared governance meetings and activities.

- » Develop subcommittees or task and work groups to engage all staff members, inter-professional and multidisciplinary team members, and even patients and families (e.g., surveys, interviews) in projects to improve care at points of service through practice and unit councils.
- » Share successes and celebrations, even small ones, with the entire staff.

- **Measuring the benefits and success** of practice and unit councils and shared governance models at points of service:
    - » Examine data collected from chart reviews, surveys, and performance measures
    - » Collect and analyze unit data
    - » Use dashboards or scorecards to display data; communicate data findings and changes to practice related to those findings in practice and unit council meetings
    - » Identify changes in practice related to data collected (e.g., Index for Professional Governance scores, Index for Professional Nursing Governance scores, patient satisfaction, employee satisfaction, quality indicators)
    - » Benchmark and measure effectiveness of practice programs based on data
    - » Provide concrete feedback to staff for their competencies and clinical practice
    - » Report findings and applications to practice to all direct-care providers and other staff

- **Evaluating and restructuring the practice or unit council may be necessary** whenever the current structure is no longer effective; there are significant changes in staffing mix, patient populations, or service leadership; or organizational redesign causes physical changes in the practice or unit infrastructure (e.g., merging two units and reducing the number of direct-care providers working on the newly reconfigured unit). Follow these steps:
    - » *Build an effective team.* The roles of providers and teams in shared governance are multifaceted and cover a wide range of activities. Creating an effective team is key to building and managing professional, multidisciplinary teams at points of service. Take these steps to ensure an effective program:
        - Assess current team functioning
        - Discuss potential positive and negative outcomes for implementing shared governance at the practice or unit level and what this means to the team
        - Note how implementing and advancing shared governance will reduce the negative outcomes (e.g., increased time and effort needed to establish and participate

in shared decisional processes) and maintain or increase positive outcomes (e.g., shared leadership) of how the team is currently functioning in terms of practice, quality, and competency

» Discuss what has to be done differently to engage in shared governance

» Identify strategies to best support and engage in shared governance:

- To reduce negative or increase positive consequences
- To engage in the new behaviors
- To develop the characteristics of an effective team

Characteristics of an Effective Unit or Practice Team

Ideally, the following characteristics will make sense to the team and fit the unique tasks, resources, and organization policies and procedures relevant to the responsibilities and accountabilities of each member of the team (according to his or her scope of practice and job description). If not, the team must address the inconsistencies to build a more effective team. This is essential if team members are to participate in shared decision-making equitably.

NOTE: *Not all decisions are shared. At times, managers and supervisors may have to direct or assign a task or activity or point out a boundary that cannot be breached organizationally. At such times, these are decisions already made by others and are only for information and compliance by the employee. However, this information may also bear on other decisions by the practice or unit council and team members and is important to building an effective team (see Appendix 32, council team-building through training and integration of health providers at points of service).*

Effective leadership

- Practice or unit council chair or designated leader accepts responsibility but does not dominate team
- Leadership may shift, depending on the issue—transformational, servant leadership, evidenced
- It is not about control but how to get the job done
- Decisions that cannot be resolved at unit level are directed to the central (governance) council(s) as appropriate (see Appendix 13, central governance council consult)
- Managers and supervisors usually take an advisory role and support the processes of shared decision-making through proactive scheduling and communication with staff and practice and unit council leadership

- Providers usually contribute by supporting initiatives in the practice or on the unit; communicating with managers and supervisors, staff, and practice or unit council members; facilitating council attendance; and managing resistance and change

Conducive work environment

- Managers and supervisors help set the climate for practice and unit shared governance
- Support shared governance at points of service
- Combination of formal and informal activities
- Mutually respectful interactions among physicians, nurses, pharmacists, and other team members
- Professional, autonomous environments of care
- People are interested and engaged

Clarity and acceptance of tasks and goals

- Clear, understood, and generally accepted
- Participative, not autocratically directed or assigned without staff input
- Everyone participates
- Everyone knows what they are supposed to do or not do
- Clear assignments are made and accepted
- Managers and supervisors ensure staff attendance, participation, and accountability by providers and staff involved in the practice or unit council and other councils and committees
- Monitor activities and progress; report progress, benchmarks, deadlines, and outcomes as they occur (see Appendix 33, sample activities in progress form)
- Managers or supervisors and staff participate in strategic planning through practice or unit councils and department or division and organization committees
- If there are questions, a contact person(s) is available

Carefully considered decisions

- Clear and determined in a way that team members are in consensus and willing to support them (see Appendix 4, sample council shared decision-making tool)
- Persons who oppose the decision will speak up or notify the practice or unit council chair or other(s), as appropriate, depending on the reason for the disagreement
- Use disagreements to explore other options, concerns, or possible consequences to ensure the final decision is the best one

- If disagreements are outside of issues related to practice, quality, competency, practice or unit operations, or boundaries (e.g., personnel issues), managers or supervisors may advise and guide councils how to best proceed
- If immediate disagreements cannot be resolved, the team leader may need to table the discussion or decision until further information and support can be obtained

Constructive feedback
- Active listening with reflective feedback
- Constructive, consistent, clear
- Peer reviews conducted consistently and according to policy (see Appendix 22, sample peer evaluation)
- Individually: as needed—there should be no surprises or bundled complaints
- Unit: provide a report of activities at least quarterly to nurse manager and all unit staff (see Appendix 31, sample council quarterly report form)
- Ongoing reports to managers and supervisors at interprofessional and multidisciplinary team meetings, assemblies, town hall meetings, and central governance council meetings when appropriate (e.g., improvements in performance measures and quality indicators reported to the central governance quality council)

Self- and group-advocacy
- Become comfortable with risk management and confronting team members with potential problems that can result in medical errors and impact nurse and patient safety
- Creatively problem solve and resolve and manage conflict (see Appendix 34, sample conflict management worksheet)
- Accept responsibility for mistakes and near misses and intervene to maintain or reestablish employee and patient safety
- Provide regular in-services and support for ethical practice among healthcare providers
- Recognize and protect (see Appendix 35, healthcare providers' bill of rights in shared governance)

Once you have established the unit- or practice-level council for engaging in shared governance at points of service, it is important to consider other stakeholders, including leadership, union partners, community members, and patients. What, then, are the roles of these stakeholders when implementing shared governance at the organization level?

Chapter 5

Implementing Shared Governance at the Organization Level

No significant learning occurs
without a significant relationship.
    —James Comer, MD

The Roles of Shared Governance Stakeholders

A consortium of stakeholders is needed to participate in shared governance for it to succeed: researchers, administrators, service executives, direct-care providers, interprofessional and multidisciplinary team members, patients, and community members. Their roles are as diverse and interrelated as their expertise, experiences, and education. Four such stakeholders (or partners) include leadership, union representatives, community members, and patients.

Leadership partners

Shared governance helps those in leadership positions—administrators, service executives, managers, and supervisors—to step back from many tasks and decisions about practice, quality, and competency that direct-care providers are more than qualified to make. Service leaders provide a professional practice environment that supports and facilitates direct-care provider autonomy.

Shared governance and case management models promote professionalism through peer and managerial relationships. All healthcare providers (e.g., nurses, physicians, pharmacists, and social workers) are potential leaders, actively engaged in influencing to achieve results so employees can practice partnership, equity, accountability, and ownership. Many providers serve as managers, or problem solvers. Management is directed toward goals, structures, processes, and resources (human, material, and fiscal).

Nurses have been key stakeholders and primary leaders in implementing shared governance within healthcare organizations and practice settings. The table in Figure 5.1 describes the differences between management and leadership and how each one impacts shared governance design, implementation, outcomes, and sustainment.

Union partners

Although a union is a complex system with many guidelines and regulations, the simplified purpose of the union in most healthcare organizations is twofold:

1. To provide collective bargaining to help employees gain control over their practice and accomplish professional and economic goals, objectives, and outcomes

2. To offer protection from demanding and unfair management standards that threaten the quality of care delivery or negatively impact the professional practice environment (e.g., unsafe or ineffective staffing ratios, mandatory overtime, and unsafe or hostile work environments, among others)

Even though both collective bargaining and shared governance are about giving providers a voice in decision-making in ways that impact practice at points of service and organizationwide, shared governance is not collective bargaining. Shared governance is a shared decision-making process.

The goal in shared governance is to integrate collaborative practice into the professional practice environment through shared decision-making. By partnering with the union representatives in the healthcare organization from the beginning of implementation, the interprofessional and multidisciplinary team members can communicate this intent and address concerns and issues as they arise, thereby increasing understanding and reducing or eliminating the confrontation that sometimes occurs in such discussions (Porter-O'Grady, 2004, 2009c).

Community partners

Healthcare providers who are engaged in shared governance partner with members of their communities in activities that reflect positively on the organization and their service, discipline, and profession. They share in the decision-making around which activities to support and to offer. Community collaborations include those with direct-care providers participating in outreach programs, such as:

- Offering a first aid or CPR training day for community members each year
- Presenting a health fair annually with direct-care providers negotiating the vendors and activities for various patient populations from the community and their families (e.g., prostate cancer screenings, smoking cessation programs, and disaster preparedness activities)

| FIGURE 5.1 | From management to leadership |

MANAGEMENT	LEADERSHIP

• **Management** – a functional process that includes interpersonal and technical aspects through which organizational goals and objectives are accomplished
• Associated with *competence* (what one knows or can do); applies learned knowledge, skills, and abilities to address situations and events in which they are sufficient to meet challenges and goals
• Transactional form (command-and-control; parental role) of managing others; informing and directing behaviors, work and services
• Use the power model of leading; role may be awarded, appointed or assigned; focuses on maintaining systems and processes
• Approach followers to exchanging one thing for another; manages contingencies
• Gatekeeping; often assume roles of critics or experts towards shared governance:
   – Intellectual wheel spinning
   – May retreat into "research"
   – Too little preparation for and willingness to undertake tasks of building better organizations in an imperfect world
   – Often sees issues, problems, or concerns as residing *out there* and not *in here*
   – Potential responses to growing staff empowerment in shared governance:
   – *Positive*: encourage greater involvement and effort by staff; create opportunities to share in decisions; provide coaching and support
   – *Negative:* threatened by perceived loss of power and influence with increased challenges; build restrictions and rules; rigidly defined roles and tasks
   – Task-driven, even when staff divided into team structures
   – Communication is often informational and uni-directional (one-way) from manager to staff
	• **Leadership** – an empowering process with underlying motivation that directs goal-oriented behaviors (choice of decision-making style used to meet a specific goal); *influencing* others to follow
	• Associated with *capability* (how one adapts to change, generates new knowledge, and improves ability and performance); enables others to adapt and face challenges using newly learned knowledge, skills, and abilities
	• Transformational form (shared, or distributed; adult-to-adult interaction) of leading others; building partnerships
	• More complex but more potent
	• Cannot be awarded, appointed, or assigned; leadership comes only from influence
	• Tolerates and builds on mistakes (*i.e.*, failing forward)
	• Discovers potential motives and goals
	• Engages the full person
	• Serves others with head, heart, hands, and habits through empowerment and shared accountability, ownership, and partnership
	• Builds relationships of mutual stimulation and elevation
	• Service first
	• Shared governance requires transformational leaders at all levels
	   – Engaged
	   – Recognizes the importance of implied and intuitive knowledge and skills
	   – Flatter, decentralized structures
	   – Centralization of programs and budgets
	   – Integrative work arrangements
	   – Team-driven infrastructures and work groups (*e.g.*, cross-functional, high-performing teams)
	   – Expanded personal and professional multi-directional communication networks

© 2014 HCPro

- Obtaining affiliations with local universities and colleges for healthcare providers (e.g., physicians, nurses, pharmacists, social services, chaplains) to continue their academic educations on hospital grounds
- Allocating and using appropriate resources to support various projects (e.g., a junior internship program that brings high school students into the organization during the summer and teaches them how to communicate with patients)

Patients as partners

Patients today are very knowledgeable and unwilling to be unilaterally directed in their treatment plans. They want a voice in what treatment approaches will be implemented, which medications they will take, and even where they will be hospitalized. Shared governance is an integrating structure that pulls all participants together: nurses, physicians, interprofessional and multidisciplinary team members, patients, and family members. As a process structure of partnership between direct-care providers and patients, shared governance provides a vehicle for improved communication, greater responsibility and accountability, and a way of coordinating, integrating, and facilitating care at points of service that is relationship-based and patient-focused.

Patients respond positively when direct-care providers partner with them in their care decisions. Some providers make walking rounds during shift changes and intermittently throughout their shifts. They stop to speak with their patients each time and ask for their feedback, questions, concerns, and ideas. If the physician came by earlier, for example, nurses might ask the patient what was said and listen to his or her report instead of telling the patient what the physician wrote in the chart or had told the nurse. These direct-care providers invite patients who are able to do so to attend the interprofessional and multidisciplinary team meetings when the team members are discussing that patient's care.

Engaging patients in conversation is one method of involving them in their own care. When direct-care providers interact relationally with patients in partnership, patient and employee satisfaction scores increase.

Healthcare providers as partners in systemswide shared governance

Healthcare providers' roles in whole-systems shared governance are multifaceted, occurring within multiple levels of the organization (i.e., macro, meso, and microsystems):

- Shared governance is a universal process structure or model. It can be applied in any setting. As it emerges in one department or division, it begins to affect members of other services, departments, and disciplines who want to participate in decisions that affect their future and roles, and who want to be involved to the fullest extent possible as shared decision-making applies to them. Such is to be expected and anticipated.

- Other departments and disciplines should be implemented when they are ready. Although nurses generally lead the process change, shared governance will vary in terms of organizational application. When other departments are ready, nursing must be ready to assist, to encourage, and to act as role models, sharing the information and experiences gathered in their own implementation process. Allow the shared governance process model to materialize in the divisions, disciplines, and departments that seek it. (See Figure 2.3: Porter-O'Grady's interdisciplinary shared governance model, 2009c.)

- Structure corporate and organizational integration into the shared governance process. Service support provides an opportunity for the organization to integrate everyone's growth in shared governance. Healthcare organizations can only manage change strategically if the whole organization joins together and providers collectively undertake the necessary structures for change together. Shared governance needs to be incorporated so it becomes an organizational imperative and continues to grow across the organization.

- When assessing whether or not shared governance is present and working, it is helpful to identify personal characteristics of how stakeholders influence others when engaging in decision-making, problem-solving, and other relational activities (see Appendix 36, influencing style interview tool).

Many organizations have developed institutional process models in which all disciplines and departments have some role in making decisions that affect the direction and operations of the organization. As individual disciplines and divisions do their work, they integrate with this larger process model (see Figure 2.4, interdisciplinary shared governance workflow chart). Every employee has an important role in the organization as a whole, participating in the directions, policies, decisions, and objectives that set the organization on a course for its own future. Healthcare providers have opportunities to lead their respective organizations into that future through shared governance.

Shared governance process models and institutional models take on a number of different designs and are directed, in essence, to provide a framework so members, divisions, and departments of the whole organization can participate together in seeking goals and objectives that guide their future. It is important that departments and divisions with such models emerge and begin to lead the future direction of the whole organization in providing a framework for integrative process models and shared decision-making.

Shared governance should be an *integrating structure,* then, that pulls all the participants together. It is a structure of partnership between manager or supervisor and staff, between organization and discipline, between division and profession, and between worker and organization. It provides a vehicle for change, ownership, equity, investment, partnership, accountability, and for a way of coordinating, integrating, and facilitating the work of healthcare today and tomorrow.

A fundamental aspect of shared governance is the need to join all of the parties together in a venture to which they are all committed. The structural process and the emergent system is part of the design for a shared governance framework that will provide an integrative structure for collectively moving the organization toward desired outcomes. This is what needs to be done to lead strategic change.

The next step in the implementation of a shared governance process is to continue gathering information and resources to design, implement, and evaluate your own shared governance process. Although there is no single right approach or process model, the basic principles and competencies of shared governance are generic, viable, and measurable.

Chapter 6

Measuring Shared Governance

Contributing author: Robert G. Hess, Jr., PhD, RN, FAAN

> *Additional problems are the offspring of poor solutions.*
> *—Mark Twain*

Andrea, an emergency room nurse, felt overwhelmed. Her chief nursing officer had just promoted her to a newly created position of shared governance coordinator. She told Andrea to go forth and implement shared governance, which was expected to be a major component in the hospital's application for the American Nurses Credentialing Center (ANCC) Magnet Recognition Program® (MRP) status that was planned for next year. Andrea's anxiety stemmed from the fact that she had no idea what shared governance was, and none of the articles she had read explained the concept in a way that a real nurse could understand.

Definitions, assessments, and measurements of shared governance are folded in a history of vagueness, stretching from its initial conceptualization and implementation to subsequent evaluation. Anthony (2004) provides an overview of this complex organizational ambiguity. Dating from its roots—when Luther Christman, PhD, RN, FAAN, spoke to the possibility of an autonomous nursing organization within a hospital at the 1975 American Nurses Association convention in Atlantic City, New Jersey—anecdotal accounts and research studies have attempted to connect shared governance with rosy outcomes. But without defining and measuring its underlying concept, governance, how can organizations assess how much of what is being *shared*, if anything at all? And if shared governance is not defined and measured, how can it be connected to competencies or outcomes?

Shared Governance: Research and Instruments

Assessments and measurements of shared governance process models range from case study exemplars and implementation stories to research-based studies. Anthony (2004) provides an excellent overview of many of these studies. A comprehensive list of published research and graduate projects can be found on the Forum for Shared Governance website. (See the bibliography in Appendix B for many additional resources and references related to shared governance structure, processes, and outcomes.)

Exemplars and case studies with subjective evaluations of outcomes provide anecdotal evidence of processes and provide a road map for designing and monitoring governance structures. An 86-item measurement instrument (Hess, 1998) was developed and validated to evaluate the distribution of governance. This tool demonstrated then and now that shared governance can be quantified so it can be connected to outcomes and competencies. Anything else is suspect.

Shared governance is an organizational innovation that gives healthcare professionals control over their practice and extends their influence into administrative areas previously controlled only by managers and supervisors. Governance models are becoming evidence-based because we are doing the research. At this point, Hess' tools have had extensive use by other researchers; the Index of Professional Nursing Governance (IPNG) has been used to measure governance in healthcare organizations for more than 20 years. The IPNG evaluates the implementation of innovative governance models and tracks changes in governance. The more global index, the Index of Professional Governance (IPG), measures the perceptions of all healthcare professionals within an organization and is realizing similar outcomes.

Clavelle, Porter-O'Grady, and Drenkard (2013) recently conducted a national study using the IPNG and Aiken's Nursing Work Index (Revised) to study the relationship between shared governance and the nursing practice environment in MRP organizations. The investigators found that in MRP organizations the primary governance structure was shared governance, which was significantly and positively related to an improved professional practice environment.

Hess organized a multigenerational group of healthcare professionals in 2013 to identify and recommend changes in the language of the indexes of professional governance instruments' items. After all, the language was more than 20 years old. Result:

- The essence of the items remained the same, therefore preserving integrity of the IPNG and IPG for longitudinal studies.
- The language of the 2.0 versions of both professional governance instruments more accurately reflect current healthcare environments and are more meaningful to today's healthcare professionals.

While there are growing numbers of tools to measure qualities and characteristics of governance, they are limited in their application across organizations and within services. The indexes of professional governance, the IPNG and IPG (see Appendix A, and Appendixes 1 and 2 in your downloads), remain the only valid and reliable instruments for measuring shared governance in healthcare today. Let's take a closer look at those instruments.

IPNG and IPG: Quantitative Measures of Governance

The IPNG is specific to nursing, whereas the more global IPG is generic for all healthcare disciplines and services. The two indexes are the first and only quantitative measures of governance and its distribution among groups within healthcare organizations (Hess, 1998, 2013). These survey instruments use 86 items to measure the balance of power, relying on a view of organizations as both rational and natural emergent systems described by the sociologist Alvin Gouldner (1959).

In his classic analysis, Gouldner related the rational view of organizations as orderly formal structures with members who pursue the achievement of the acknowledged goals of the organization. This is the entity defined in organizational charts. However, an alternate organization, the natural or emergent organization, often exists outside of those charts. Natural structures emerge within an organization from groups with informal power that is hard to ignore. These groups sometimes pursue goals and agendas that are more relevant to them as professionals and not always aligned with the goals of the organization.

Specifically designed for nurses, the IPNG:

- Relies on the perceptions of the people surveyed within an organization to report not only which group has official authority over certain areas, but also which group has control and influence beyond the recognized and accepted order.
- Provides a baseline assessment of which groups have control and influence over vital organizational areas, such as professional practice and the resources that support it, before innovative organizational governance models are implemented. The survey tool can track changes in key areas during implementation, validate implementation, and provide benchmarks against other organizations.
- Compares governance scores of groups (e.g., management and staff, specific units and practices or departments) within the organizations and provides guidance for those on the MRP journey.
- Offers the first opportunity to connect changes in governance to professional, clinical, and organizational outcomes across all micro- (unit- or practice-level), meso- (departments or divisions), and macrosystems (organizations).

During the past 20 years more than 150 organizations, nationally and internationally (i.e., in several facilities in Lebanon and Jordan), have used the indexes of professional governance to evaluate the implementation of innovative management models and to track changes in governance. More than 35 MRP-status hospitals have used the IPNG to evaluate their progress in developing and establishing shared governance *(http://sharedgovernance.org/?page_id = 158)*.

The IPNG is currently the most respected and frequently used measurement instrument for evaluating shared governance. It is included in ANCC's shared governance toolkit (Haag-Heitman and George, 2010), Swihart's books on shared governance (2006, 2011), and the shared governance practice brief distributed to executives in member hospitals by the Advisory Board Company (2005), a think tank based in Washington, D.C. The IPNG appears in more than 75 reported research studies. The vast majority of the research and evaluation assess shared governance in single settings, using either cross-sectional or longitudinal time frames. (See notes at the end of this chapter on using these tools.)

Although no other instruments purport to measure governance across organizations, a few hospitals have created homegrown surveys to track implementation progress at their own institutions. Others have authored instruments that measure concepts closely related to governance. For example, Havens created a governance-related instrument, the Decisional Involvement Scale, to measure actual and preferred decisional involvement of staff nurses and managers on nursing units (Havens and Vasey, 2003). Implementing a shared governance practice model changes the organizational culture. Shared governance moves any organization from a hierarchical structure in any form to a practice- or unit-level (practice- or unit-based), councilor, administrative, or congressional structural form that requires ongoing interprofessional collaboration, communication, flexibility, evaluation, and redesign of goals and processes.

When and How to Measure

The decision to assess the state of governance in an organization cannot be made lightly. Surveying staff brings up questions of confidentiality, confidence, and comfort. Surveys can even be threatening to some, depending on the environment and how specific information can seem to participants. For example, while practice- or unit-specific information can be important for strategic planning or targeted intervention, identifying practices and units with just a few staff members can be viewed as compromising their anonymity. Some organizations may discover scores they had not anticipated, while others may find their expectations validated.

Related literature and consultants alike are unclear about when and how often to assess or evaluate process or progress. Generally, the best time to assess governance is before implementation or revitalization of a program, and again after a vital change has been affected.

Most organizations measure change at about two-year intervals. One hospital assessed governance before implementation of a shared governance model and then annually thereafter. The administrators and staff put a lot of energy into their program. The scores validated the slow but steady progress of governance maturity. After a few years, survey scores demonstrated the organization placed firmly in the zone of shared governance.

Measuring governance with the IPNG before or during implementation can guide the creation of a strategic plan and refinement of the model. By tracking 86 individual items, participants can often identify those items with scores that can be improved on most easily and quickly within their particular organizational environments. Targeting items for change amounts to "teaching the test" because the items define governance. Changing them advances the resulting overall governance score.

Research on the Evidence and Principles of Shared Governance

Destiny is not a matter of chance, it is a matter of choice;
it is not a thing to be waited for, it is a thing to be achieved.
—William Jennings Bryan

For those interested in learning more about the research and work done over the past 30 years on shared governance and leadership, excellent articles and books are available from the fields of business, management, economics, human resources, and healthcare. Nurses and interprofessional partners completed multiple studies in 2013 (see Appendix 37, samples of 2013 research on shared governance articles). The research continues to grow as investigators implement the IPNG and IPG instruments to measure shared governance. For example, Walter, Aucoin, Brown, Thompson, and Sullivan (2014) used the IPNG instrument to evaluate clinical nurses' participation and engagement in shared governance when looking at the role shared governance plays in engaging them in evidence-based practice.

Anthony, Hess, Porter-O'Grady, Swihart, and others have studied the principles of shared governance and found them to be accurate delineators of empowerment (Anthony, 2004; Howell et al., 2001; Porter-O'Grady, 2003a, 2003b, 2004, 2009a, 2009b, 2009c; Swihart, 2006, 2011). They and their colleagues have investigated multiple theoretical and empirical evidences to define shared governance and to determine whether or not a shared governance practice model based on the principles of partnership, equity, accountability, and ownership achieves the positive outcomes desired.

An important research project conducted in 2001 by J. N. Howell, Frederick, Ollinger, Hess, and Clipp looked at shared governance in a government agency using the IPNG measurement tool. Let's see why it was so important.

Research on shared governance in a government agency

In a landmark study at the Durham VA Medical Center in North Carolina, Howell and his colleagues (2001) used the IPNG to study an established shared governance process model within a government agency, a highly bureaucratic and hierarchical organizational management system. They defined nursing governance as:

> ... *multidimensional, encompassing the structure and process through which professional nurses in healthcare agencies control their professional practice and influence the organizational context in which it occurs ... [and] loosely described shared governance as a system of structuring nursing practice that gives nurses at the bedside the responsibility for decision related to their practice. In the words of Prater, it implies the allocation of control, power, or authority (governance) among mutually (shared) interested and vested parties (pp. 187–188).*

Six dimensions for measurement

The researchers studied 183 registered nurses (RN) in nursing service at the Durham VA Medical Center (273 surveys were distributed but only 183 [67%] returned). They used the 86-item IPNG instrument to measure nurses' perceptions of professional nursing governance facilitywide on a continuum ranging from *traditional* (dominant group is nursing management/administration) to *shared* (decision-making shared between direct-care nurses and management/administration) to look at the following six dimensions with sub-scales:

1. **Nursing personnel:** Who controls nursing personnel by hiring, promoting, evaluating, recommending, adjusting salaries and benefits, formulating unit budgets, creating new positions, conducting disciplinary action, and making terminations?

2. **Information:** Who has access to information relevant to governance activities, such as opinions of managers, staff nurses, physicians, patients, and interdisciplinary team members; unit budgets and expenditures; nursing service goals and objectives; and the organization's finances, compliance reports, and strategic plan?

3. **Goals:** Who sets goals and negotiates the resolution of conflict at different organizational levels among nurses, other members of the interdisciplinary healthcare team, and organizational leadership, as well as philosophy, goals, objectives, and a formal grievance procedure?

4. **Resources:** Who influences the resources that support professional practice: monitoring and securing supplies, recommending and consulting other services, determining daily assignments, and regulating patient movements (admissions, transfers, referrals, placements, and discharges)?

5. **Participation:** Who creates and participates in committee structures related to governance activities, such as committees that address policies and procedures for clinical practice, staffing, scheduling, budgeting, and collaboration?
6. **Practice:** Who controls professional practice in terms of patient-care standards, standards of professional practice and care, quality, staffing levels, qualifications, competency, professional development and education requirements, and evidence-based practice (incorporating research into practice)?

Higher scores on any of these six sub-scales indicated staff nurses perceived themselves to have greater influence over professional decision-making in their organization. Scores for three of the six dimensions (nursing personnel, information, and goals) were consistent with a traditional governance environment, although the scores on information and goals were very close to the shared governance range. In the other three dimensions (participation, resources, and practice), nurses perceived a significant shift toward shared governance with scores near or higher than the base range for shared governance.

The results of this study demonstrated that "shared governance within several critical areas of nursing practice can be successfully implemented" within an organizational structure thought to be traditional and bureaucratic (Howell et al., 2001, p. 195). This study demonstrates that shared governance can be implemented in any organization or practice setting, although the degree to which it is implemented and its characteristics may be shaped by each unique environment. Shared governance can and will look different in every organization.

Further research using valid and reliable instruments such as the IPNG have begun to examine outcomes associated with varying levels of implementation of shared governance and its role in the recruitment and retention of nurses. As medical care is integrated into healthcare systems, community-based outpatient centers, and cyber technologies that triage and treat patients across cyberspace, staff nurses are becoming more involved in shared decision-making. The indexes for professional governance provide critical guidelines for measurement. Questions yet to be considered more fully include:

- What impact will shared governance have on the professional practice environment of care for new generations of healthcare providers in a socio-technological era?
- What competencies and standards of practice are emerging as shared governance is folded into the fabric of organizations?

As shared governance transforms nursing practice, the IPG is being used to assess physicians' and allied health professions' involvement in shared governance in hospitals, as well as commercial entities involved in healthcare. Even patients have begun to sit on councils and participate in shared governance.

Research on measuring shared governance

For many additional resources and references related to seminal and current research done on shared governance structure, processes, and outcomes with the use of the indexes for professional governance (IPNG and IPG), see the bibliography in Appendix B. A comprehensive list of published research and graduate projects can be found on the Forum for Shared Governance website, *www.sharedgovernance.org*.

NOTE: *Using the IPNG and IPG—The sub-scales keys are necessary to interpret the indexes for professional governance (IPNG and IPG). Although they are proprietary, they are available at no charge to researchers, clinicians, and administrators who formally request permission and agree to adhere to guidelines for use and reporting.*

Chapter 7

Interprofessional Shared Governance in Healthcare

The Interprofessional Approach

Contributing authors: Susan R. Allen, PhD, RN-BC; Dawn Nebrig, MSW, LISW; and Jennifer K. Munafo, MA

This chapter offers an introduction and description of influences in building interprofessional shared governance (IPSG) structures in healthcare organizations.

> *In a real sense all life is inter-related.*
> *All men are caught in an inescapable network of mutuality, tied in a*
> *single garment of destiny. Whatever affects one directly affects all indirectly.*
> *I can never be what I ought to be until you are what you ought to be,*
> *and you can never be what you ought to be until I am what I ought to be.*
> *This is the inter-related structure of reality.*
> —Martin Luther King, Jr.

An interprofessional approach to shared governance must be embedded throughout the organization adopting it, from the clinical decisions at points of service to the strategic priorities placed on interprofessional issues by senior leadership. A cornerstone of this approach to practice may be the inclusion of patients and families as full partners on both care teams and planning groups. Respecting and valuing the knowledge and service of all team members contributes to a trusting, openly communicative, learning environment and positive patient care and practice outcomes.

Collaboration is critical for direct and indirect patient care and among disciplines on interprofessional committees, councils, and task forces. Whether to improve an existing process or to develop strategic new initiatives, an interprofessional team represents the best collaborative effort. With this approach to care and decision-making, each unique need and perspective is captured to enhance outputs and improve outcomes. Some of the influencing factors on a more pervasive approach to shared governance include the following:

- Interprofessional governance in healthcare organizations
- The American Nurses Credentialing Center (ANCC) Magnet Recognition Program® (MRP)
- The Institute of Medicine's (IOM) reports on the healthcare environment

Let's take a closer look at these three factors as they relate to IPSG.

Influences on Interprofessional Governance

The healthcare environment has experienced dramatic changes since shared governance was first introduced more than three decades ago. Similarly, forces impacting care delivery systems influence organizational governance structures. Neither top-down authoritative nor discipline-specific structures alone can be sufficiently effective in an environment requiring engaged and collaborative partnerships among all of the individuals responsible for providing healthcare services.

A foundational principle of shared governance states those who do the work of the organization must share in decisions about their work to arrive at the best decisions. Today's care environments present an immediate need to improve patient safety and clinical outcomes while increasing the efficiency, effectiveness, and timeliness of how care is provided across service lines. Decisions must be made rapidly and accurately in response to these calls to action. In short, the governance structure for decision-making should reflect the current and evolving demands of an increasingly interprofessional care delivery system. IPSG is such a structure.

ANCC Magnet Recognition Program®

The MRP components of structural empowerment and exemplary professional practice delineate expectations for direct-care nurses' involvement in the governance of healthcare organizations (ANCC, 2014). MRP organizations are required to have generally flat, flexible, and decentralized governance structures. Nurses at all levels in these hospitals and healthcare systems must be involved in decision-making relative to their practice, competency, quality, and team-based patient-care delivery systems. There must be evidence of shared governance structures and processes to establish standards for nursing practice, address concerns of nurses, and support their professional development. The MRP program also expects nurses to demonstrate participation and leadership in interprofessional teams to positively impact patient care and clinical outcomes.

IOM reports on the healthcare environment

Few things have had a greater impact on the values, beliefs, and cultures of healthcare organizations than the series of reports published by the IOM over the past 11 years (IOM, 2000, 2001, 2004, 2011). Each of these well-researched publications looked deeply at the causes of problems in healthcare systems. They exposed devastating outcomes, including the frightening reality that nearly 100,000 lives are lost annually due to errors or negligence in care delivery in the United States (IOM, 2000).

The first report, in 2000, suggested a need for a comprehensive approach to improving patient safety, with new legislation, governance structures, strong leadership, performance standards, and expectations to reduce medical errors (IOM, 2000).

In 2001, the IOM proposed six major aims and the 10 simple rules for healthcare in the 21st century to improve the timeliness, equity, effectiveness, patient-centeredness, efficiency, and safety of care. These six major aims, though simple to state and impossible to disagree with, were not common in the cultures or structures of U.S. healthcare organizations. The 10 rules, which begin with "care based on continuous healing relationships," and contain the concepts of "shared knowledge," "clinician cooperation," "patient in control," and "anticipation of needs," among others, were viewed as critically necessary but not the current reality of hierarchical, physician-dominated healthcare (IOM, 2001).

In its third report, the IOM (2004) called for transformational leadership to resolve patient safety problems in the work environment and advocated for improved working conditions related to staffing and scheduling. Improvements were also needed in work processes and workplace design to improve communication and efficiency to reduce errors and waste. Shared decision-making between management and staff were to be valued and become the expectation for standard practice (IOM, 2004).

However, nursing's professional position was not strengthened until 2011, when the IOM published its report on the importance of nurse roles in healthcare delivery and the need for dramatic changes in their work environments. This report stated that nurses should practice to the full extent of their licenses and become equal, interprofessional partners with doctors, pharmacists, and other members of the healthcare team. More important, nurses must become leaders in healthcare, leading change to advance health. IPSG creates a structure and culture within healthcare organizations, setting the stage for necessary improvements in clinical outcomes, care delivery systems, and multidisciplinary communication.

Case Study: Cincinnati Children's Hospital

Cincinnati Children's Hospital, in Cincinnati, Ohio, is one of the largest children's hospitals in the United States, with 625 inpatient beds and emergency, psychiatric, outpatient, and urgent care services delivered in 16 locations throughout its tristate region. We believe our shared governance structure is currently effective and continuing to grow as a strong, viable decision-making structure. However, this was not always the case.

Shared governance history and original structure

Cincinnati Children's has had a nursing shared governance structure in place since 1989. Following the integration of allied health professions with the Division of Nursing in 1995 to become the Department of Patient Services, a second interdisciplinary structure for allied health professionals was developed and implemented in 1999. The word *interdisciplinary* was chosen rather than *multidisciplinary* because we believed *multidisciplinary* indicated there were multiple coexisting disciplines but did not convey the sense of interaction we desired between disciplines. Our two governance structures operated in parallel, with few occasions for interface and little collaboration (see Figure 7.1).

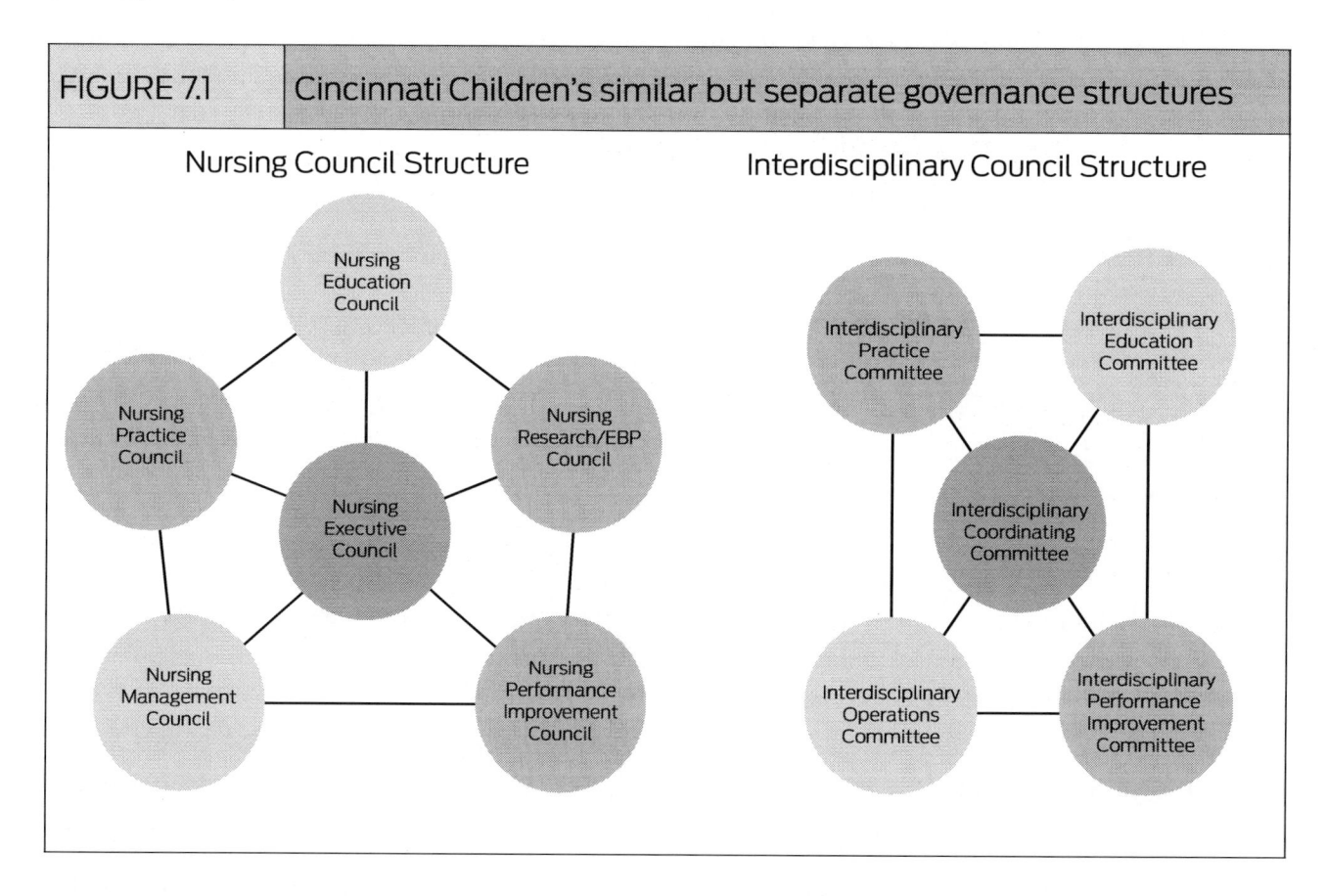

FIGURE 7.1 — Cincinnati Children's similar but separate governance structures

Nursing Council Structure:
- Nursing Executive Council (center)
- Nursing Education Council
- Nursing Research/EBP Council
- Nursing Performance Improvement Council
- Nursing Management Council
- Nursing Practice Council

Interdisciplinary Council Structure:
- Interdisciplinary Coordinating Committee (center)
- Interdisciplinary Education Committee
- Interdisciplinary Practice Committee
- Interdisciplinary Operations Committee
- Interdisciplinary Performance Improvement Committee

This two-silo structure was characterized as being inefficient, cumbersome to navigate, and unclear in its roles and responsibilities (Hoying and Allen, 2011). Because of these inefficiencies, the overall governance structure in patient services had weakened over time. In 2002, we significantly increased the frequency of interprofessional initiatives, collaborations, and systems-improvement work following the selection of Cincinnati Children's as one of the recipients of the Robert Wood Johnson Foundation Grant to pursue perfect patient care.

By spring 2005, the increase in collaborative practice precipitated discussions during which the purpose and efficiency of the two separate structures were considered. As the frequency of interprofessional collaboration grew, the need for interprofessional decision-making became an imperative. Questions arose about the purpose, effectiveness, and viability of maintaining two governance structures. The patient services operational and shared governance leadership began the work of merging the structures to better reflect our new interprofessional reality (Hoying and Allen, 2011).

Implementation: Enhancing shared governance

Our Interdisciplinary Coordinating Council (ICC) and the Nursing Executive Council (NEC) joined forces in 2006 to begin efforts to integrate the shared governance structure. This combined group was named the Shared Governance Enhancement Team. This team met regularly over the next two years to create an integrated and efficient decision-making structure for optimal patient outcomes for the Department of Patient Services. Councilor structures were established for decision-making about broad interprofessional issues that impacted multiple disciplines centrally, profession-specific practice decision-making within each discipline, and decision-making by the interprofessional teams who practiced at the points of service.

Over the next two years, the team worked diligently to create an integrated governance structure that promoted efficient decision-making around issues relating to interprofessional and profession-specific practice for optimal patient outcomes. Consensus was reached on eight critical elements of an effective shared governance structure:

1. The shared governance structure must be integrated—no silos.
2. Shared governance is the hub of decision-making—shared governance is connected and a player in the work of the organization.
3. Shared governance work has defined, visible, and measurable outcomes.
4. Meaningful work is done in shared governance councils and committees.
5. Managers create the environment for shared governance.
6. The shared governance structure is easily articulated: streamlined, efficient, and effective.
7. There is representation of all patient services members in the shared governance structure.
8. Shared governance is integrated deeply into our culture; there is excitement about shared governance.

Using these guiding principles, a proposed model revision was developed and shared with patient services direct-care providers and managers for input and feedback. Consultative assistance was sought from nationally recognized shared governance leaders, Timothy Porter-O'Grady, DM, EdD, ScD(h), FAAN, and Vicki George, RN, PhD, FAAN. Their recommendations included:

- Streamline the current interdisciplinary divisional structure into one interprofessional council for decision-making about systems issues that cross professions; interprofessional practice, education, and research issues would be on this agenda

- Ensure each profession with representation on the interprofessional council has a profession-specific governance structure

- Design the structure to promote decision-making closest to points of service

As the work to create the new structure progressed, regular updates were shared by the representatives of the shared governance enhancement team. Feedback was sought using a variety of communication strategies, and was incorporated until agreement was reached on the new structure. Our enhanced Interprofessional Shared Governance Council structure was launched July 2008.

Evaluation: Nurse and allied health perceptions

Prior to the launching of the enhanced Patient Services Shared Governance Structure in 2008, a research study was conducted in February 2007 to determine the nursing and allied health professionals' current perceptions of shared decision-making. We used Dr. Robert Hess' 1998 Index of Professional Governance (IPG) tool. The IPG tool (Hess, 2013) is described in detail in Chapter 6, and is provided in the downloads for this book.

Baseline data were collected on the then-current perceptions of shared governance in patient services. A total of 631 individuals (32% of the eligible staff) completed this survey. In 2007, the total sample mean score of 170.0 (SD 59) indicated registered nurses and allied health professionals felt there was room for improvement in shared decision-making. IPG values indicating shared governance range from 177 to 352. The study was repeated in November 2010, two years after the enhancement launch in 2008, to gather data to compare differences in the perceptions of shared governance from 2007 to 2010. The 2010 study goal was to use the resultant data to guide the continued enhancements to Cincinnati Children's shared governance interprofessional structure.

Multivariate analysis of variance was conducted to simultaneously test if IPG sub-scale scores changed from 2007 to 2010, and if there were differences between nursing and allied health responses. In 2010, 947 individuals completed the tool—a response rate of 33.5%. The 2010 total sample mean score of 178.6 (SD 61) showed the nurses and allied health professionals now perceived shared decision-making was occurring. Changes from 2007 to 2010 were significant in the nursing and allied health professionals' total Governance Scores, and in the Participation and Goals Scale Scores. No other significant changes or interactions were noted (Hoying and Allen, 2011).

Cincinnati Children's interprofessional structure and responsibilities

The IPSG model (see Figure 7.2) is designed around the Cincinnati Children's mission of practice, education, and research. All levels of the Cincinnati Children's shared governance councils include direct-care providers, managers, and other professionals with roles that are essential in contributing to informed decision-making of the council members.

For example, educators are members of each of the discipline-specific and point-of-service education councils, in addition to the direct-care provider and management representatives. All of the chairs and chairs-elect of the councils are direct-care providers.

1. **Professional discipline governance structure**
   Each profession is responsible for decisions about practice in their discipline-specific shared governance structure. All participate in the interprofessional governance structure. These professional disciplines include: audiology, child life, integrative care, nutrition therapy, nursing, occupational therapy, pharmacy, physical therapy, recreational therapy, respiratory therapy, social work, and speech pathology. Each profession has a council structure that is responsible for the accountabilities of professional practice, education, inquiry (research, quality improvement, and evidence-based practice), and coordination of the discipline's shared governance activities.

2. **Point-of-service governance structure**
   At the points of service, IPSG councils are responsible for decision-making about the care provided for specific patient populations. Cincinnati Children's calls these the "Point-of-Care" councils. Chaired or cochaired by a registered nurse, these councils review professional practice, education, research, and evidence associated with the specific patient populations.

3. **Patient Care Governance Council (PCGC)**
   The PCGC is a systemwide interprofessional council made up of the chairs of every profession. It started meeting monthly in March 2008. Although the higher purpose of shared decision-making was described in the Interprofessional Shared Governance Council Charter, the actual meetings were typically information-sharing only. Sharing information about Cincinnati Children's safety reports and employee engagement surveys accomplished the goal of linking direct-care providers and clinicians to organizationwide initiatives and strategic priorities, but did not empower them to make decisions about interprofessional practice.

   PCGC's information-sharing format changed when the opportunity to develop an interprofessional practice model (IPM) surfaced. A review of the nurse practice model prompted the question, "Could this model apply to all professions?" Professions reviewed their professional practice standards and determined there were no regulations or standards prohibiting them from practicing within an interprofessional practice model. PCGC then assumed the responsibility for developing the model. Shared purpose, mutual commitment to the benefits of the outcome, and profession-specific structures for reviewing and approving recommendations moved the model development forward. The 12-month facilitated process resulted in an IPM that sets the standards for team-based care throughout patient services (see Figure 7.3).

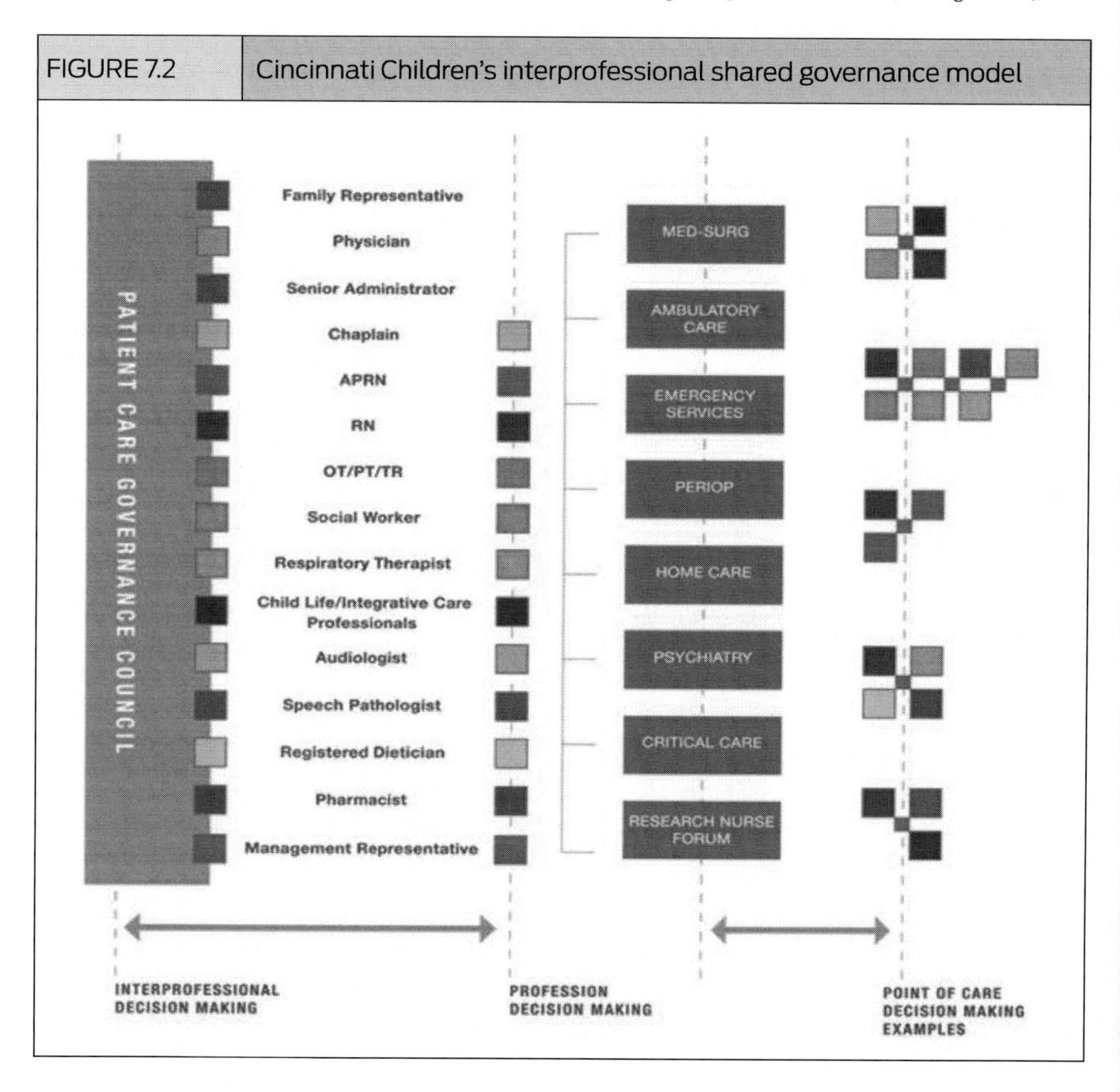

FIGURE 7.2 — Cincinnati Children's interprofessional shared governance model

Patient Care Governance Council members:
- Family Representative
- Physician
- Senior Administrator
- Chaplain
- APRN
- RN
- OT/PT/TR
- Social Worker
- Respiratory Therapist
- Child Life/Integrative Care Professionals
- Audiologist
- Speech Pathologist
- Registered Dietician
- Pharmacist
- Management Representative

Profession Decision Making areas:
- MED-SURG
- AMBULATORY CARE
- EMERGENCY SERVICES
- PERIOP
- HOME CARE
- PSYCHIATRY
- CRITICAL CARE
- RESEARCH NURSE FORUM

INTERPROFESSIONAL DECISION MAKING | PROFESSION DECISION MAKING | POINT OF CARE DECISION MAKING EXAMPLES

FIGURE 7.3 Cincinnati Children's interprofessional practice model

Gears labeled: Safety, Comprehensive Coordinated Care, Innovation & Research, Best Practice, Professionalism, Collaborative Relationships — Working Together for OPTIMAL OUTCOMES

© 2013 Cincinnati Children's

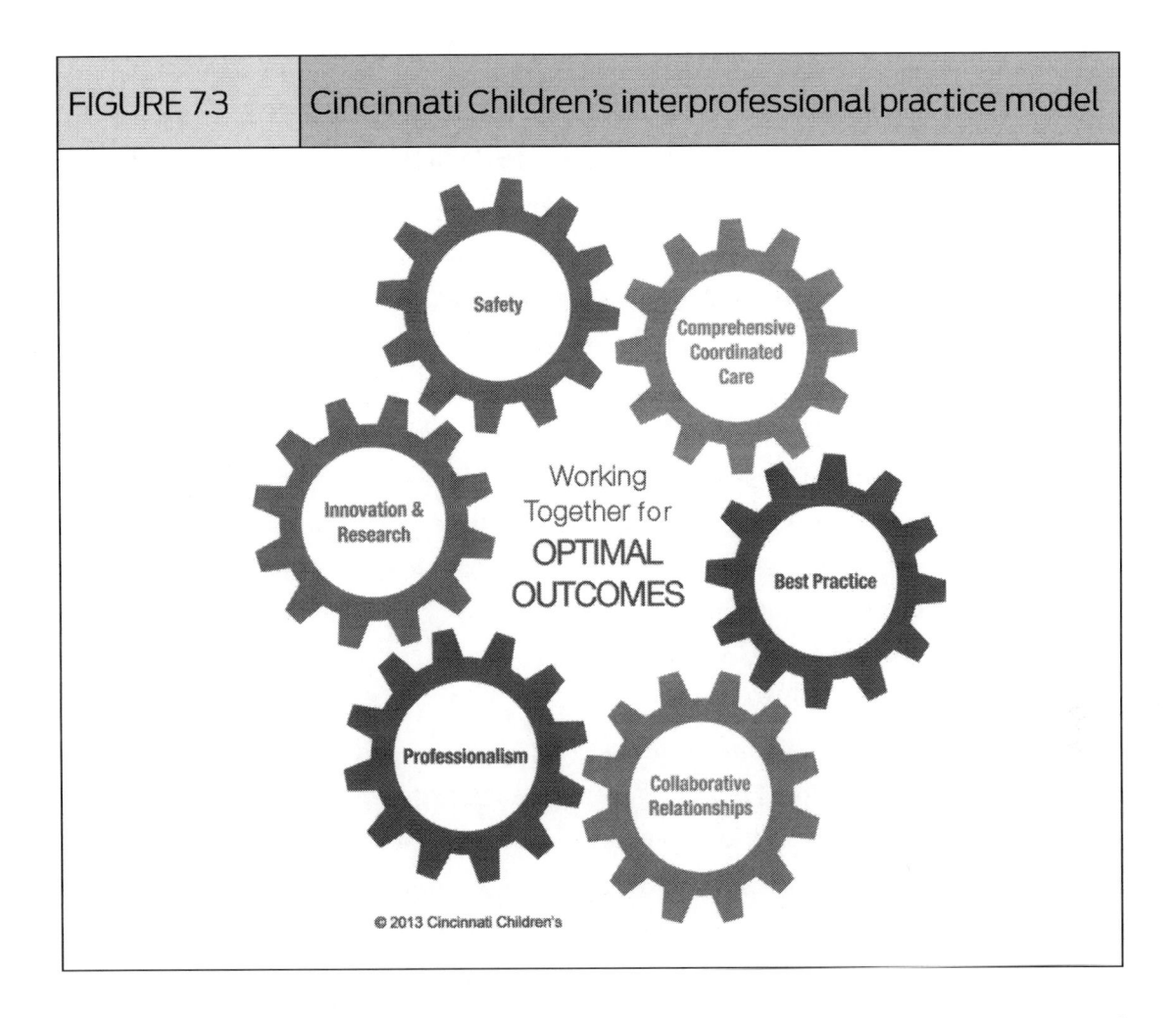

The PCGC makes decisions regarding professional practice, professional education, and professional inquiry concerns that span across professions and are systemwide in scope. It is the highest-level council in Cincinnati Children's shared governance structure. Each discipline has its own shared governance structure and each discipline is represented on the PCGC, as is the interprofessional management council chair, for example. The PCGC also includes members from both the medical governance structure and chaplaincy services, as well as family representation from Cincinnati Children's Family Advisory Council. Dr. Cheryl Hoying is the Patient Services Leadership and Senior Administrator representative on PCGC.

4. **Nursing shared governance**

As noted earlier, nursing shared governance is the oldest and most mature of Cincinnati Children's governance structures. A brief description of the structure may be helpful to understand our decision-making processes. Due to the large number of nursing professionals at our organization, there are four decision-making levels to enable the participation of direct-care nurses within the nursing shared governance structure:

    a. *Point-of-Care Councils (Interdisciplinary).* Daily decisions start at points of service. A point-of-care council is defined as "an interprofessional group of direct-care providers and managers who practice with a shared patient population and in a common geographic location." The membership of point-of-care councils represents the professions who provide care in that practice environment. In most areas, these councils are chaired or cochaired by a nurse.

    b. *Nursing Cluster Coordinating Councils.* There is one nursing cluster coordinating council for each defined cluster. (See Figure 7.4.) Clusters are made up of direct-care nurse coordinating council chairs from points of service in similar care areas. Cluster councils enable nurses to make decisions that impact practice across like units, such as critical care, inpatient medical-surgical care, ambulatory care, emergency and urgent care, home care, perioperative care, psychiatry, and research.

5. **Nursing profession divisional councils**

    There are three professional nursing governance councils and the Nursing Profession Coordinating (Executive) Council. The professional nursing governance councils are as follows:

    a. *Nursing Professional Practice Council.* Ensures nursing practice results in the delivery of safe, high-quality, evidence-based care.

    b. *Nursing Professional Education Council.* Provides direction for the Division of Nursing's professional education and development to ensure delivery of safe, high-quality, evidence-based care.

    c. *Nursing Professional Inquiry Council.* Ensures an environment of scholarly inquiry to support provision of safe, high-quality, and evidence-based care.

    d. *Nursing Profession Coordinating Council.* Sets priorities for shared governance work within professional nursing councils, ensuring alignment with strategic initiatives of the organization and coordination of councils for optimal outcomes.

FIGURE 7.4	Cincinnati Children's nursing cluster coordinating structure		
Med-Surg	Ambulatory Care	Peri-Op	Psychiatry

• Adolescent Med/Surg (A6N)
• Complex Airway (B5CA)
• Complex Pulmonary (A7C1)
• CRC/Diabetes/Sleep (A7C2)
• General/Community Medicine (A6S)
  • Neuroscience/Pediatric Medicine (A7N/S)
  • Rehabilitation (A4C1)
  • Transitional Care (A3S)
  • GI/Colorectal Surgery (A4S)
  • Complex Surgery/Solid Organ Transplant (A4N)
  • Observation Unit (Liberty)
  • Short Stay (A3N)
  • SRU
	• Primary Care: Adolescent Med, Teen Health, PPC, PCF, Hopple, Batesville, Mayerson
	• Allergy, AERO, Pulmonary
	• IAC, IDC, Derm, Ophtho, ENT
	• Neuro, NSurg
	• Plastics, Peds Surgery, GYN, Colorectal, HVMC
	• Rheum/Rehab
	• Sports Med, Ortho
	• Neph, Urology
	• GI
	• Cardiology
	• DDBP, Genetics, Pain
	• Endo/Diabetes
	• Complex Care, DPIC, EB
		• Short Stay (A3N)
		• Fetal Care (A7FC)
		• Interventional Radiology
		• Anesthesia Imaging
		• OR – Burnet
		• PACU – Burnet
		• SDS – Burnet
		• Infusion Center
		• Periop Liberty
		• VAT
		• Cath Lab
		• Wound Care
			• Medical (A4C2)
			• Residential (P2E, P2S, P2N)
			• Inpatient Latency (P2W)
			• Inpatient Adol (P3N & P3W)
			• Inpatient Child (P3S)
			• Neuro-Psych (P3SW)
			• Lindner Center of Hope

Emergency Services	Home Care	Research Nurse Forum	Critical Care
• Emergency Department • Transport Team	• Private Duty Nursing • Agency • Liaisons • Starshine Hospice	• CTO • TRTO • CTRC • Divisional	• Hem/Oc/BMT/IPU (A5S/N/C) • Cardiac Step Down (A6C) • CICU (B6HI) • Dialysis (A1) • NICU (B4) • PICU (B5CC) • SRU

Breaking down silos
Demonstrable benefits to our interprofessional governance structure

Building a culture of interprofessional team-based collaboration means we must break down long-established silos. Those silos have deep roots that foster mistrust through misunderstanding associated with our profession-specific training and socialization. IPSG is worth implementing because, through the process and structure, professions learn from each other. We spread best practices and stretch perceived boundaries using the examples of professions that have already crossed them. There is improved coordination of resources, and allied health professionals benefit from effective nursing structures. Synergies emerge. We have recognized opportunities for interprofessional collaboration in professional development, education, and research.

One fundamental premise of our shared governance environment is that for the best decision-making to occur, those directly working in that area of practice must be involved in decision-making about that practice. A second major premise of our shared governance philosophy is that the majority of decision-making about practice should be occurring at the point of service. By actualizing these two premises, nurses and allied health professionals from all settings and roles are empowered to actively participate in all levels of organizational decision-making groups at Cincinnati Children's. We anticipate continuing the spread of our improved integrated governance structure.

A unique opportunity we are currently exploring is the inclusion of the PCGC chair on the medical executive committee. It is profound when existing decision-making structures seek out partnerships with leaders of IPSG. Work has been initiated on our next chapter at Cincinnati Children's, the integration of IPSG with organizational decision-making structures beyond patient services where it makes sense to do so.

Looking back
Deconstructing our formula for interprofessional shared governance

With the benefit of hindsight and learning from integrated IPSG activities, we have reflected on what we now consider essential elements to our success. Listed below are lessons learned throughout our journey, the importance of which we did not fully appreciate in their moments. We hope our insights may help your organization avoid some of our struggles, and more fluidly move your efforts forward with greater effectiveness and efficiency. These are some of the essential elements we discovered for successful implementation of IPSG:

1. A clear and unequivocal expectation from the senior vice president/CNO that each profession develops its own shared governance structure to govern practice. Leveraging the traditional hierarchy's top-down authority provided directors of all professions with the acceptance and

support they needed to move forward to allocate resources and set the vision for their respective professions. Including directors in our consultation sessions with Drs. Porter-O'Grady and George helped them partner with their clinical leaders in designing their profession-specific structures. Each of the 11 allied health professions was at a different place along the continuum of shared governance implementation. Therefore, the design team had to include a clinical representative from each profession and engage the management leader from each profession. A clear delineation of the intended destination provided the necessary direction to sustain a journey with few predetermined milestones.

2. Commitment to and comfort with the iterative nature of the design process. If there were a "foolproof cookie cutter," we would have used it. The trust, goodwill, and partnership that developed through the shared process forms the foundation for our interprofessional structure. The first step was to bring together stakeholders to represent (or who were connected to) all areas implicated in the team's decision-making processes. We quickly learned to involve leaders from whatever shared governance structure existed and vet recommendations through established councils. If shared governance was new to allied health disciplines, those disciplines developed a process for discussion among the clinicians who would now be part of the organization's shared governance. Our enhancement process took two years, causing some turnover in membership; we added new members as gaps in representation were identified. Although these changes might be considered interruptions, we actually benefited from the reflection points such transitions created. We also learned the process needs to be as transparent as possible. We posted the design team meeting minutes to our intranet and routinely requested input from existing councils.

3. A nimble interprofessional structure standardizes principles and encourages customized practice. Early in our process we wasted time trying to build an interprofessional structure before we fully identified our underlying principles. Following our consultation with Drs. Porter-O'Grady and George, we stepped back and came to consensus about what the principles of shared leadership would be at Cincinnati Children's (see Figure 7.5).

Once the shared leadership model was established, each profession was able to design the structure they needed to meet identified accountabilities. Some professions designed a single coordinating council structure; others designed a multicouncil structure. All structures have the same general accountabilities for professional practice, education, inquiry, and coordination. Furthermore, professions continuously evaluate the goodness-of-fit of their customized structures to achieve the standard accountabilities with the greatest effectiveness and efficiency.

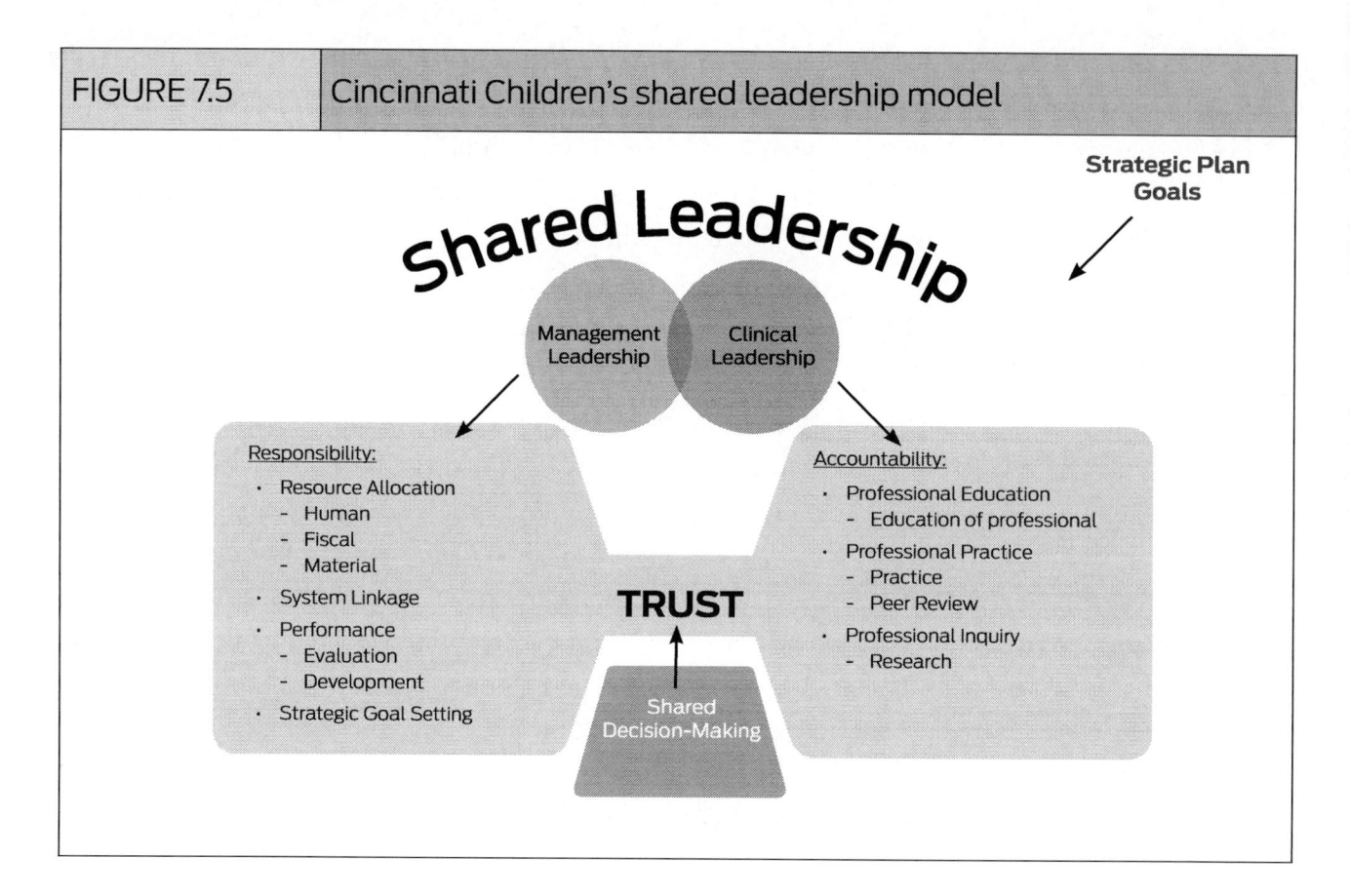

FIGURE 7.5   Cincinnati Children's shared leadership model

Shared Leadership

Strategic Plan Goals

Management Leadership   Clinical Leadership

Responsibility:
- Resource Allocation
  - Human
  - Fiscal
  - Material
- System Linkage
- Performance
  - Evaluation
  - Development
- Strategic Goal Setting

Accountability:
- Professional Education
  - Education of professional
- Professional Practice
  - Practice
  - Peer Review
- Professional Inquiry
  - Research

TRUST

Shared Decision-Making

Shared governance requires ongoing support and development. We found that each year as new nursing and allied health members join the councils at divisional and points-of-service levels, it is imperative to our own success to continue to provide education and training. Our basic education for successful council leaders includes the following topics:

- *Shared Governance 101* introduces and contextualizes the four basic principles of shared governance (accountability, partnership, equity, and ownership) into the culture and organizational structure of Cincinnati Children's Hospital.

- *Meeting Management* outlines the steps to preparing for, leading, and project managing the work of shared governance council meetings. Designing outcomes-oriented agendas and minutes is a fundamental skill taught during this session.

- *Role Clarification* delivers concrete expectations and responsibilities for each member role on councils and includes a full discussion of the benefits of and techniques for decision-making by consensus.

- *Goal Setting* provides a simple formula for identifying meaningful council goals that are practice-driven, connected to organizational strategic priorities, and measurable.

The half-day education sessions are offered multiple times throughout the day and evening shifts to accommodate our direct-care providers' schedules. Education helps ensure staff members are able to engage in and sustain shared leadership—the outcome of shared governance. Managers are also members and encouraged to attend training sessions to help them build their partnerships with the council chair, to further understand their role in council participation and mentorship, and to provide a management perspective through interprofessional dialogue during the skill-building session.

Dedicated facilitators are needed to sustain and grow a viable IPSG. Success is not guaranteed because a governance structure was designed. You cannot cross your fingers and hope the vision will be realized. Prior to the launch of our interprofessional structure in July 2008, we anticipated this potential problem and requested—and received—funding in the patient services operating budget for two full-time shared governance facilitators. These facilitators directly support 21 councils (PCGC, Interprofessional Management Council, eight allied health coordinating councils, four housewide councils, and seven cluster nursing councils). They provide "as needed" support to all point-of-service councils and council-sanctioned subcommittees and work groups. The shared governance facilitators at Cincinnati Children's support the principles of shared governance theoretically and logistically. The principles of accountability, partnership, equity, and ownership are safeguarded because the facilitators ensure a shared mental model for shared governance across professions, points of service, and throughout the organization.

Facilitator support includes coaching and mentoring through agenda planning, meeting facilitation, meeting debriefing, and consultation with chairs and key stakeholders involved in issues before the council when needed. Our facilitators encourage open dialogue and share what works within the structure to support intra- and interprofessional growth. They have position descriptions that describe their facilitator responsibilities (see Figure 7.6).

In summary

Creating an environment in which governance is truly shared is not an easy thing to do and requires the ongoing commitment and attention of all members of the organization. Sharing governance requires significant changes in the culture of an organization and in the behaviors, beliefs, and values of its members. A few false assumptions such as the following may challenge your progress:

- If we have shared governance councils, we have shared governance
- If we have multiprofessional councils, we have interprofessional decision-making
- If shared governance is interprofessional, nursing will lose its voice

These concerns must receive focused time and ongoing attention throughout IPSG design, development, training, and implementation. IPSG has immeasurable benefits for an organization, its members, and all internal and external stakeholders. Consider these words from a nursing shared governance council chair—who did not lose her voice—as she describes her experiences with IPSG:

> *All the right people are at the table, from bedside nurses to pharmacists, to physicians, to educators, to … everybody coming together for the mutual purpose of seeing if this idea is feasible and beneficial and productive … I see so much more of an emphasis on the team, and on the understanding that it is the team that makes the difference. It's not the individual components thereof. That's what shared leadership is; it's the engagement of everybody (Allen, 2013).*

FIGURE 7.6	Cincinnati Children's facilitator responsibilities
Facilitation	Description: Facilitates teams and groups with a specific focus and intent to ensure attainment of goals and reinforce accountabilities of the team members to their respective roles. May plan, organize, and design meetings or work sessions. May drive consensus and build cohesiveness to achieve performance and results.
Leadership, Advocacy, and Ethics	Description: Promotes and provides guidance, resources, and knowledge for professional growth across the organizational level and in the community. Acts as a champion for education by creating a dynamic learning environment and cultivating a culture of lifelong learning supporting individuals in their own professional development and learning processes. Serves in key roles and influences decisions at the system level through participation on committees, councils, and task forces. Evaluates own practice in relation to ethical principles. Identifies and addresses ethical issues within the learning environment. Mentors peers and others when situations arise that create ethical conflicts. Engages in honest and ethical behavior by role modeling and assisting others in understanding ethical behaviors.
Collegiality, Collaboration, and Consultation	Description: Partners with subject matter experts and other leaders to enhance quality and usefulness of education programs. Demonstrates effective resource management. Uses effective teaching, coaching, and mentoring behaviors that help others reach their full potential. Seeks opportunities to be taught, coached, and mentored. Establishes collegial partnerships contributing to the professional development of peers, students, colleagues, and community to affect change and generate positive outcomes. Facilitates active involvement and complementary contributions of others in team meetings and discussions. Seeks and employs diverse resources when appropriate to optimize outcomes. Provides direction and consultation to enhance the abilities of others to learn and impact change at the system level.

We have illustrated how IPSG came to be, and is in place and thriving at Cincinnati Children's Hospital, where we are proudly committed to the delivery of safe, quality care through an interprofessional approach to shared governance. This interprofessional philosophy is embedded throughout the organization, from the clinical decisions at points of service to those from the Interprofessional Patient Care Governance Council to the strategic priorities placed on interprofessional issues by Senior Vice President of Patient Services and Chief Nursing Officer, Dr. Cheryl Hoying.

From the early days of her tenure at the medical center, Dr. Hoying worked to ensure systems were in place and properly supported for shared decision-making. Our principal supportive structure for the participation of nurses, other care providers, and leaders from all roles and settings in decision-making is the IPSG structure. We strongly believe including people impacted by decisions will result in better decisions, actions more widely supported across services, and empirical outcomes sustained over time. The why of what needs to be accomplished is communicated to and realized by everyone involved in the work of the organization. IPSG gives direct-care provider's ownership of their practice at every point of service across the organization.

Chapter 8
Case Studies

Snapshots of Shared Governance in U.S. and Global Communities

> *If the infrastructure does not consciously bring the teams together on an ongoing basis to build their relationships and to integrate their practice, partnerships will not be created, and the duplication, repetition, and fragmentation of care will not stop.*
> —Bonnie Wesorick

Shared governance takes on different constructs in various organizations because of the unique culture of each institution. However, if organizations remain true to the principles in their design, implementation, and evolution, then they share the basic elements, or attributes, of shared governance—they are just rolled out in different ways.

This chapter details the inner workings of shared governance in two vastly different hospitals. Consider how the process is similar despite the differences in size, settings, locations, and cultures.

Case Study 1

Beaumont Hospital, Royal Oak, Michigan, USA
Contributing author: Anne Ronk, RN, MSN, NEA-BC
Nursing Director of Women, Children's and Psychiatric Services

Background

Beaumont Hospital is a 1,070-bed tertiary care academic medical center that employs more than 2,000 registered nurses in Royal Oak, Michigan. The Beaumont Royal Oak health system leadership model is described as physician-led, nurse-partnered, and administratively supported. Nursing has always had an integral role in the organization, but the decision-making structure within the division of nursing needed to be transformed.

Beaumont Royal Oak had implemented shared governance in the early 1980s. More than 20 years later, a Professional Nurse Council (PNC) was created to provide each unit the opportunity to interface with hospital nursing leaders. The council was primarily a communication vehicle for the nurses and consisted of approximately 80 bedside staff nurses, two nurse managers, and one director of nursing. Some units had councils that had remained active from the original structure, but other units had allowed their councils to cease functioning.

In 2011, a new chief nursing officer (CNO) was hired. She quickly identified a need to create more engaged and empowered nurses. While the PNC had served a valuable purpose, it became evident to her the forum was too large and unwieldy for effective decision-making. The unit-level councils also needed to be reenergized.

Redesigning shared governance

With support from the CNO, 15 nurse representatives began meetings in February 2013. Staff nurses from the PNC, managers, clinical nurse specialists, and an administrator discussed changes needed to truly facilitate the mission and vision of Beaumont Royal Oak with and for nurses.

This newly formed PNC redesign team met every other week for nearly a year and a half to create and roll out the new shared decision-making processes and governance structure. Their activities included:

- Assessing our current governance structure
- Researching and reviewing nursing governance structures to identify best professional practices, i.e., reviewing research articles and exploring other hospitals' shared governance models
- Interviewing and emailing representatives of hospitals with strong shared governance models, such as:
    - » Kim Derr, director of staff development and research at Akron (Ohio) General Hospital. In our discussion regarding evaluation of a shared governance program, Kim suggested we consider looking at the Hess tool. Akron General was in a similar situation in redesigning their shared governance.
    - » Stacey Brull, director of nursing research, informatics, and Magnet Recognition Program® at Mercy Medical Center in Baltimore, Maryland. We examined her shared governance program development and three-year longitudinal study.
    - » Jamie Ezekielian, James Comprehensive Cancer Center (JCCC) at Ohio State University in Columbus, met with our entire professional nurse council via conference call and responded to questions and shared much appreciated information.

Following our calls with JCCC, we arranged for the redesign team members to travel to Columbus, Ohio, in October 2013 to meet with key leaders of their shared governance and leadership team, who presented a comprehensive review of their shared governance journey and program. They discussed their bylaws and professional practice model. Breakout sessions gave leaders and staff nurses opportunities to speak with their peers and explore specific topics pertinent to their practice. Going forward, we used what we learned (e.g., we referenced the JCCC bylaws in our new documents).

During one of our redesign team meetings, we found the Forum for Shared Governance and decided to reach out to Robert G. Hess, Jr., RN, PhD, FAAN, the founder. Dr. Hess (Bob) responded with enthusiasm and answered many questions for us. We received his permission to use the Index of Professional Nursing Governance (IPNG) instrument to measure where we were in establishing shared governance.

The IPNG, an 86-question survey, measures nurses' perception of governance on a continuum from traditional decision-making to shared governance to self-governance. It has been used and validated by healthcare systems across the country. The survey is broken into six dimensions of governance: access to information, resource influence, personnel control, and decision-making related to practice and strategic planning. Results are classified in three categories:

- Traditional governance (management dominant)
- Shared governance (dominance can be primarily managerial or primarily staff, but always shared between the two)
- Self-governance (staff dominant)

We sent the survey out to every single registered nurse at Beaumont Royal Oak, hoping for at least a couple hundred responses. The response was much greater. The survey was first taken by the PNC representatives during their scheduled meeting. Then surveys were sent electronically to all nurse staff members and left open for two weeks. The results were used as a baseline measurement of staff's opinion of where we were in building shared governance and how it is viewed in the health system. Another survey will be sent out when our new model is complete and then again three years afterward to trend our progress.

Of the 1,108 nurses who began the survey, 899 completed it. The response represented 66 different cost centers within Beaumont Royal Oak, of which 28 units had more than 50% of their nurses complete the survey. Therefore, the results successfully reflected our nurses' perceptions, giving us confidence in the findings. The overall score fell in the primarily management-dominant shared governance category. However, 78% of the nursing units surveyed fell into the traditional management-dominant category for governance. Only one of the six dimensions of governance fell into the category of shared governance: the influence-over-resources dimension. This survey validated the PNC redesign team's assessment.

Beaumont Royal Oak now had an opportunity to move the existing governance model to one where staff nurses would be more involved in every type of decision made going forward.

We then consulted with Diana Swihart, PhD, DMin, MSN, CS, RN-BC. Dr. Swihart reviewed our redesign team minutes and project work. She met with the director liaison to the group via a conference call. During the call, Dr. Swihart shared an idea for how to weave a connection between the Magnet Recognition Program® (MRP) standards and a shared governance structure. Drs. Swihart and Hess were then invited to present an eight-hour conference on shared governance and transformational leadership. The presentation was attended by PNC members and nurse leaders. The content included a review of the results of our survey and an overview of shared governance programs.

Implementation

As a result of our preparatory work and conference, the redesign team learned about and defined our shared governance structures and systems. We developed an organizational structure to support our shared governance model. We restructured active committees within the health system to include nursing representation.

The group then identified several key issues to address next:
- Communication of our new shared governance model
- Staff involvement with practice decisions
- Staff accountability
- Staff's and administration's understanding and awareness

Our present governance structure includes councils already in existence and new nursing governance councils we are still building. The established councils include unit-based councils, a hospitalwide professional nurse council, a nursing executive leadership council, an MRP council, and the clinical integration council.

1. Unit-based councils

Each nursing unit implemented a unit council for problem-solving and decision-making at the unit level. Each unit determined its own membership criteria and meeting times to meet the unit needs. Each unit council developed its own bylaws based on the Beaumont Royal Oak nursing mission, vision, values, and professional practice model. The unit council reviews pertinent data and information to develop action plans to resolve issues and assists the hospitalwide nursing governance councils to identify unit representatives to councils, work groups, and committees. Each unit council is expected to establish a mechanism of communication between staff, unit council, and hospitalwide councils.

2. Hospitalwide professional nurse council

This council, whose membership includes all unit council chairs, supports change and facilitates culture-shaping through mentorship and education to strengthen the framework and outcomes of all unit-based councils. The council provides a forum in which unit leaders collaborate, inspire, and support one another as they strive to deliver exceptional nursing care that exceeds the expectations of patients, families, faculty, staff, and the community. This council meets to share and gather information, as well as interface with the CNO, CMO, and CEO. The chair of the hospital professional nurse council is a member of the nursing executive leadership council.

3. Nursing executive leadership council

This council, whose membership includes all Royal Oak nursing leaders, also supports change and facilitates culture-shaping through education and information-sharing. The focus of the council is to support and strengthen the framework and outcomes of all the nursing governance councils. This council meets to share and to gather information, as well as interface with the CNO on topics critical to the profession of nursing and germane to the delivery of nursing services throughout Beaumont Royal Oak.

4. Magnet Recognition Program® council

This council has oversight and responsibility for achievement and maintenance of the American Nurses Credentialing Center's MRP. The MRP council actively works on preparation of the program application process along with promoting a culture to achieve quality indicators and nursing practice standards. It also provides related education and site-visit preparation. The council interfaces with each of the nursing governance councils in order to gain information and evidence of standard compliance. The chair of the MRP council is a member of the nursing executive leadership council.

5. Nursing clinical integration council (NCIC)

This council coordinates, integrates, and monitors the activities of the Beaumont Royal Oak nursing shared governance councils and may mediate unresolved issues within or between councils. The nursing clinical integration council (NCIC) is chaired by the Beaumont Royal Oak CNO. The purposes of the NCIC are to guide the vision and coordinate and implement the processes of the councilor system of shared governance at Beaumont Royal Oak, incorporating the core values and guiding principles of care for nursing into all decisions and activities. The NCIC acts as an official conduit for coordinating activities of all nursing governance councils (and MRP council representatives) for and in support of all nursing employees to promote and guide professional growth and competency through communication, coordination, and staff development activities around practice, quality, and competency of nursing staff.

Our revised structure includes five new nursing governance councils to serve as decision-making groups with specific authorities and responsibilities. The new nursing governance councils are: professional practice council; nursing quality and patient safety council; education and research council; operations, finance, and leadership council; and advocacy, service, and community council.

New structures and responsibilities

The nursing governance councils act as the official representative for and in support of all nursing staff to promote and guide professional growth and competency through communication, coordination, and staff development activities around practice, quality, and competency. The structure of nursing shared governance facilitates communication, collaboration, and coordination of nursing functions. Each nursing unit and area has the opportunity to involve direct-care nurses, other staff, and management personnel in the governance structure at the unit level and council level, and to influence decisions related to practice, quality, and competency.

Beaumont Royal Oak's shared governance model artistically portrays the nursing structure for shared decision-making (see Figure 8.1). This model is a subset of our larger nursing professional practice

FIGURE 8.1	Beaumont Nurse Professional Practice Model

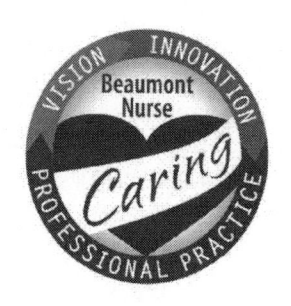

The **Beaumont Nurse Professional Practice Model** illustrates the integration of nursing practice with the mission, vision, philosophy, and values that embody the spirit of Beaumont Nurses. Our **Caring Model** is comprised of the concepts: Caring, Vision, Innovation, and Professional Practice.

Caring. Caring is the center of all we do. Caring practice includes empathy, compassion, diversity, respect, and dignity. It is a nurturing way of relating to another, toward whom one feels a personal sense of commitment and responsibility. Our **passion** for nursing is at the heart of how we deliver care and develop our professional nursing practice. We form **relationships** and **collaborate** with patients, families, and colleagues to promote optimal health outcomes in the communities we serve.

Vision. As Beaumont Nurses, we continually strive for **nursing excellence**. We are empowered through a **shared governance** model which promotes **leadership** at all levels of nursing.

Innovation. As Beaumont Nurses, we integrate **new knowledge**, **evidence-based practice**, and **research** into clinical practice and care delivery. We make visible contributions to the science of nursing through participating in research.

Professional Practice. As Beaumont Nurses, we function within the American Nurses Association's Standards of Professional Nursing Practice. We demonstrate **accountability**, **autonomy**, and **critical thinking** in our nursing practice. Continuous professional development is recognized as essential to our practice and supported through **education**, **mentoring**, and reflective learning.

Source: Adapted from resources provided by Anne Ronk (2014). Beaumont Nurse Professional Practice Model. Royal Oak, MI: Beaumont Health System. Used with permission.

model, which integrates nursing practice with the mission, vision, philosophy, and values that embody the spirit of Beaumont nurses. Our caring model is based on these four concepts: caring, vision, innovation, and professional practice. The concept of shared governance relates directly to the vision component of our nursing professional practice model. Specifically, as Beaumont nurses, we continually strive for nursing excellence. We are empowered through a shared governance model that promotes leadership at all levels of nursing.

Visualizing the shared governance model

"The Family Protected by Healing Herbs" sculpture, which has been a recognizable icon on the building's facade since the hospital's inception, was chosen as the core tenant of the shared governance model because it symbolizes Beaumont nurses' principle philosophy of "the patient is the center of all we do," including decisions that are made related to our nursing practice.

Our new shared governance model (see Figure 8.2) illustrates the Beaumont family surrounded by leaves and columns. The Beaumont family sculpture was inspired by the verse, "The leaves of the tree were for the healing of the nation."

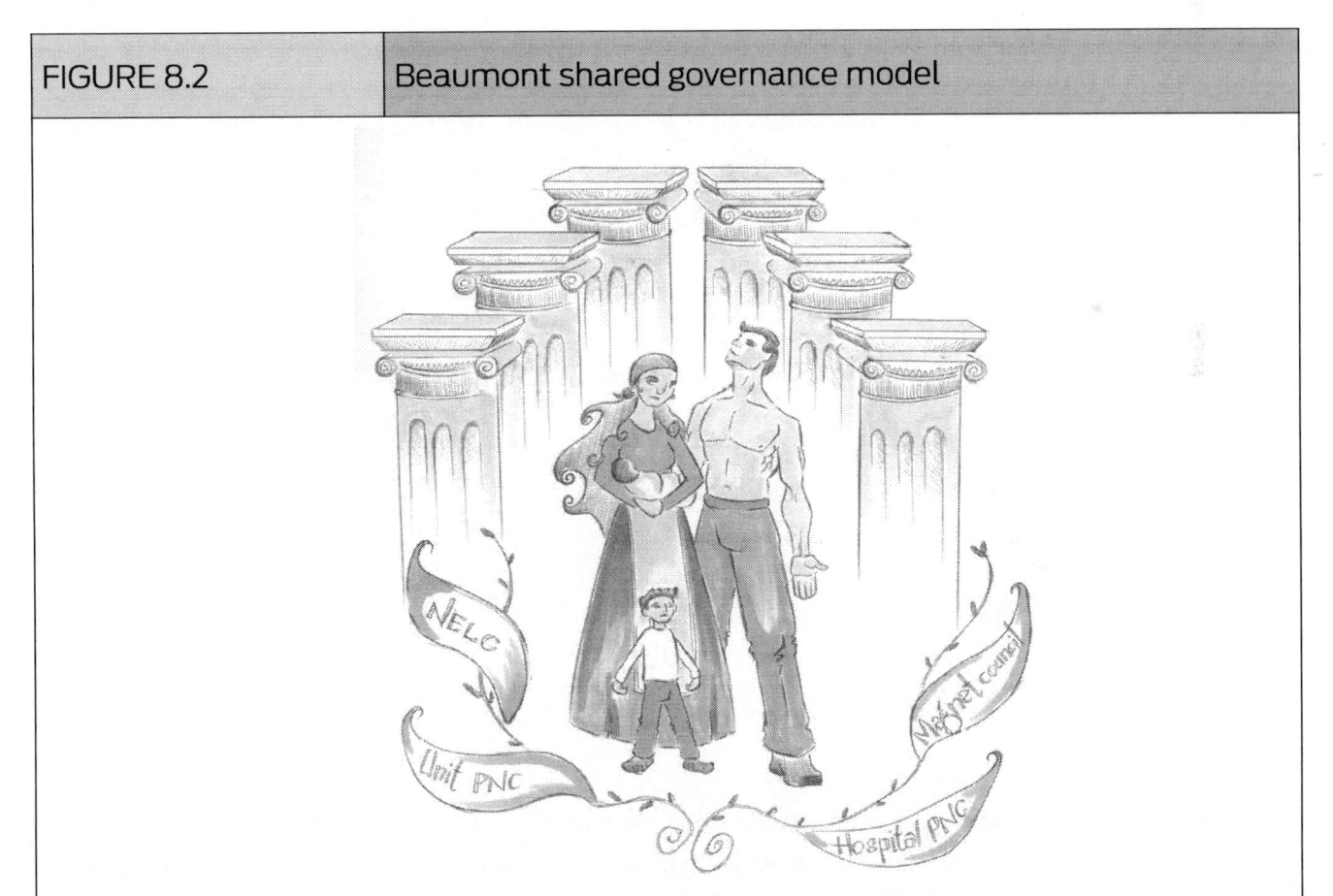

FIGURE 8.2	Beaumont shared governance model

Source: Adapted from resources provided by Anne Ronk (2014). Beaumont Nurse Professional Practice Model. Royal Oak, MI: Beaumont Health System. Used with permission.

The leaves and columns encompassing the family reminds us that nursing is involved in the governance structure at the unit level and council level, and has the power to influence decisions related to nursing practice, quality, and competency. The leaves, forming the foundation for the family, exemplify working committees that are already in existence and have membership from nursing at all levels.

The columns also have significance because they align with the strategic framework of the health system, which has five unique pillars as its foundation. The archway of columns symbolizes the clinical integration council along with these new nursing governance councils:

1. Professional practice
2. Nursing quality and patient safety
3. Education and research
4. Operations, finance, leadership, and advocacy
5. Service and community council

Each of these five nursing governance councils will include membership from direct-care nurses representing 11 different practice areas. These nursing governance councils will serve as a decision-making body with specific authority and responsibility to promote and guide professional growth and competency through communication, coordination, and staff development activities.

Beaumont Royal Oak's shared governance councilor model is based on the belief that decisions made in collaboration with direct-care nurses and nursing administration will result in optimal outcomes for patients, families, nursing, and the community. Each of the five new nursing governance councils will include membership from direct-care nurses from 11 different practice areas, administrators, clinical nurse specialists, and other individuals necessary to the functioning of the councils. The nursing governance councils will all be chaired by a direct-care nurse with the exception of the operations, finance, leadership, and advocacy council, which will be chaired by a nurse manager. We tied the roles and responsibilities of each of these councils to the MRP standards.

1. Professional practice council

Role: To define, implement, and maintain the Beaumont Royal Oak standards for clinical nursing practice consistent with national, state, and community standards of practice.

Responsibilities include but are not limited to:
- Promoting and integrating the standards of care for nursing practice, including, but not limited to American Nurses Association (ANA) standards into the Beaumont Royal Oak professional practice model

- Describing and demonstrating how nurses develop, apply, evaluate, adapt, and modify the professional practice model, caring VIP
- Establishing, reviewing, and revising policies and procedures related to nursing practice utilizing evidence-based practice (EBP) and research
- Establishing the structures and processes by which nurses are involved with evaluation and allocation of technology and information systems to support practice and nurses' participation in architecture and space design to support practice
- Participating in evaluation and development of care delivery systems to ensure continuity, quality, and effectiveness of care within and across services and settings; ensuring regulatory and professional standards are incorporated into care delivery systems
- Establishing, reviewing, and revising evaluation tools to ensure nurses at all levels routinely use self-appraisal performance review and peer review, including annual goal-setting, for ensuring competence and professional development
- Developing a peer review program, which includes reviewing and revising the process of evaluating professional accountabilities and job descriptions, and performing peer reviews, competency assessments, and performance appraisals
- Reviewing structures and processes used to improve workplace safety for nurses based on standards (e.g., ANA's Safe Patient Handling and Movement, and guidelines from The Joint Commission and IOM, among others)
- Assisting direct-care nurses to incorporate guidelines (e.g., ANA, 2005; organization and regulating agencies' approved standards for scheduling, delegation) from nursing specialty organizations and federal and state-mandated requirements into staffing and scheduling processes
- Collaborating with nursing quality and safety council to describe structures and processes including direct-care nurse involvement in tracking and analyzing nurse satisfaction or engagement data
- Promoting and recognizing nurses in attaining certification and advanced nursing education
- Advocating at the legislative level for professional practice changes, issues, and regulations by attending advocacy days representing Beaumont

2. Nursing quality and patient safety council

Role: To promote and ensure provision of highest quality and safe patient care throughout the continuum for all patients.

Responsibilities include but are not limited to:

- Developing, implementing, and evaluating an annual nursing quality improvement plan consistent with the nursing strategic plan, quality improvement goals and priorities, and state and federal regulatory agency standards
- Providing ongoing monitoring of patient outcomes in response to nursing process, continuous quality improvements, and patient safety goals
- Participating in national database(s) for data collection and measurement; using this information to facilitate prevention of negative outcomes and promotion of higher standards of care, including measurement of nursing care and related outcomes against established standards, including benchmarking with recognized external resources
- Aligning and collaborating with all nursing councils and unit councils to promote evidence-based changes, provide educational programs, and address quality, patient safety, and performance improvement opportunities
- Assisting with regulatory preparedness and compliance (e.g., The Joint Commission)
- Monitoring root cause analyses for all nursing sentinel events and adverse events to initiate improvements in practice

3. Education and research council

Role: To define and maintain educational standards promoting nursing professional development and ongoing clinical competency and quality in all practice settings for nurses at all levels through professional development, integration of evidence-based practice (EBP), and research into clinical practice.

Responsibilities include but are not limited to:

- Promoting and evaluating educational programs including, but not limited to nursing orientation, mandatory education, nursing grand rounds, preceptor education, graduate nurse residency, and professional development programs
- Defining competency measurement methodology and priorities
- Exploring potential partnering opportunities with local colleges of nursing
- Encouraging and supporting professional growth through formal presentations at local, regional, and national organizations
- Facilitating implementation of staff education through in-services, staff development programs, and continuing education (contact hours)
- Participating in educating nurses at all levels on basics of research (e.g., terminology, research methods, and the research process)
- Assisting and mentoring nurses at all levels who conduct nursing research at Beaumont Royal Oak prior to submission of their research proposals to HIC

- Increasing nursing research visibility locally, statewide, nationally, and internationally
- Encouraging professional nursing development by promoting certification, professional ladder, and academic advancement
- Participating in determining utilization of monies from the "nursing fund"

4. Operations, finance, and leadership council

Role: To facilitate excellence and promote positive patient outcomes in an environment supporting autonomous professional nursing practice in strategic planning, advocacy, influence, resource allocation, utilization, visibility, accessibility, and communication.

Responsibilities include but are not limited to:
- Developing strategies to promote culture changes that positively impact professional practice and inspire innovation
- Identifying and removing barriers prohibiting staff from having the time, resources, and energy to provide every patient with exemplary care and to participate in shared governance activities
- Guiding transitions during periods of planned and unplanned change through advocacy and influence
- Assessing, describing, and demonstrating how nursing's mission, vision, values, and strategic and quality plans reflect the organization's current and anticipated strategic priorities
- Defining and standardizing nursing roles using public health code, ANA, and other specialty nursing practice standards
- Utilizing educational methodologies to develop management skills regarding staff engagement; supporting and guiding nurse leaders as they value, encourage, recognize, reward, and implement innovation within the organization, the service, and at points of service
- Utilizing ANA Standards for Nurse Administrators and current literature to guide leadership practice
- Developing and implementing systems (e.g., Kaizen program) to achieve improved efficiencies, patient flow, and throughput
- Establishing and maintaining staffing patterns to meet needs of defined patient populations; utilizing productivity benchmarking data (i.e., NDNQI) to monitor effectiveness of staffing models
- Collaborating with human resources on recruitment and retention activities

5. Advocacy, service, and community council

Role: To coordinate, integrate, and monitor the activities of the Beaumont Health System's shared governance philanthropic activities, nursing recognition, community outreach, and patient experience and education.

Responsibilities:

- Maintaining strategies promoting excellence and recognition in nursing professional competency and quality in all practice settings for nurses at all levels (i.e. Daisy, Nightingale, Caring Spirit, Saluting Our Stars) and unit-specific recognition
- Coordinating Annual Nurses' Week recognition and activities including scholarship awards and poster sessions
- Contributing to community outreach activities and coordinating community resources (e.g., education, fundraising)
- Coordinating hospital Professional Nurse Council Legacy Committee; identifying projects; participating in fundraising, etc.
- Establishing and promoting relationships among all types of community organizations to develop strong partnerships that improve nurses' image related to their contributions to patient outcomes and health of the communities they serve
- Identifying and advancing strategies for recruitment, retention, and recognizing and celebrating achievements by nurses within the organization and community
- Reviewing patient satisfaction data aggregated at the organization level showing how Beaumont Royal Oak outperforms the mean of national databases used (e.g., NDNQI, HCAHPS, Press Ganey); this includes analysis and evaluation of data and resultant action plans at points of service related to patient satisfaction and addresses:
  » Pain
  » Education
  » Courtesy and respect
  » Careful listening
  » Response time
  » Other nurse-related national survey questions based on clinical specialty

Determining council membership

Nurses at all levels and from all departments are encouraged to participate and are governed through this shared governance infrastructure. Those interested in council membership were asked to complete a Council Membership Application and the Reference Form (see Figure 8.3).

The NCIC maintains council memberships. Applicants are responsible for notifying their immediate supervisor they are applying for council membership and obtaining the supervisor's signature on their applications. Member selection is based upon past committee experience and current participation in unit, nursing division, and governance activities, and a genuine interest in the work of the

FIGURE 8.3 Beaumont council membership application

BEAUMONT, ROYAL OAK NURSING SHARED GOVERNANCE
COUNCIL MEMBERSHIP APPLICATION

Please review the member/leadership responsibilities before completing your application. Your signature reflects that you meet the requirements and agree to fulfill the council responsibilities. Please answer the following questions in full including specific examples. You may use the back if you require more space. Next, obtain your immediate supervisor's signature and return the completed application to the Nursing Shared Governance mailbox in the Nursing Administration Office or submit the form via email.

Name (required): _____

Date: _____ Unit/Practice: _____

Preferred contact information:
Tel. Ext: _____
Email: _____
Cell Phone: _____

How long have you worked in your current position?

Please list the councils in which you are interested:

Would you be willing to consider a leadership position on the council?   Yes/No

Please list at least two references (peer/manager/colleague):
Reference 1: _____   Reference 2: _____

Why are you interested in this council position? (Please respond for each council selected. Use back if necessary.)
_____

Please share any committees you have participated in during the past 5 years and skills that you have developed which relate to the responsibilities of the council for which you are applying. _____
_____

Communication is critical to the effectiveness of the council. How will you best communicate council objectives with your peers?
_____

What strengths do you possess which will assist you in representing your clinical practice area?
_____

Applicant Signature: _____   Date: _____

Unit/ Practice: _____

Print Name: _____   Email _____

Address: _____

I am aware of this candidate's application and, if selected, will schedule off-unit time for him/her to attend council meetings or complete council assignments. I understand that if this applicant is elected for a leadership position at the executive board level, that additional time commitments will be granted. My signature further states that the applicant is not currently in a corrective action process and has received a "fully effective" on his/her most recent performance evaluation.

Immediate Supervisor: _____   Date: _____

© 2014 HCPro

council. All applicants must have effective communication and collaboration skills. A Scorecard for Council Membership Form (see Figure 8.4) was developed to be used in the selection process.

Additionally, unit-based councils needed a process for selecting a replacement council member in the event the current member is unable to fulfill the position. The nursing manager will support and facilitate the process to ensure members, or their designees, can participate in their unit-level and central governance council activities.

Ensuring staff involvement in council activities

Each nursing governance council is composed primarily of staff nurses. The chairperson for each governance council is a direct-care nurse, except for the operations, finance, leadership, and advocacy council, which is chaired by a nurse manager. This council has significant direct-care nurse membership such that decisions are still influenced by those providing care to the patients. Staff nurses are supported to attend council meetings by arranging their schedules so they can participate in meetings and complete councilor work and other activities. Direct-care nurses are compensated for the time spent in meetings and in other council work.

Developing leadership skills

Ongoing, continuing education is supported and promoted. Education is provided at each hospital-wide professional nurse council meeting on a variety of leadership topics. Hospital- and unit-based professional council members were invited to the all-day workshop on shared governance and transformational leadership with Drs. Swihart and Hess. Another all-day workshop is planned for new members of the five nursing governance councils. This workshop will provide education on meeting management, decision-making processes, program management, change management, and other leadership topics.

In addition to specific education related to leadership, staff nurses are encouraged to participate in Kaizen activities throughout the year. The Kaizen methodology of continuous improvement was adopted by Beaumont Royal Oak and has become the approach used by all staff and managers to implement incremental change. Direct-care nurses have participated in more than 80 Kaizen events. This gives nurses a solid background of experience they can draw on as they engage in shared governance activities.

FIGURE 8.4 — Scorecard for Beaumont council membership application

BEAUMONT, ROYAL OAK NURSING SHARED GOVERNANCE
SCORECARD FOR COUNCIL MEMBERSHIP APPLICATION

Application # _____

Name of Council: _____

Clinical Practice Area: _____

NOTE: For questions dealing with interest in council, past committees, communication and professional strengths, please score on a 0-2 scale.

- 0 points: None or poor explanation.
- 1 point: Limited or one example.
- 2 points: Good explanation with multiple examples.

Council leadership interest:	0	1	2
Committee participation	0	1	2
Communication skills	0	1	2
Professional strengths that applicant possesses	0	1	2
Strength of recommendation/referrals:	0	1	2

TOTAL # OF POINTS: _____

NOTES:
_____
_____
_____
_____
_____

Source: Adapted from resources provided by Anne Ronk (2014). Beaumont Health System Council Membership Application. Royal Oak, MI: Beaumont Health System. Used with permission.

| Figure 8.5 | Beaumont shared governance organizational overview |

Top-level councils: Quality and Patient Safety | Education and Research | Professional Practice | Operations/Finance and Leadership | Advocacy Service/Community

Other entities: Magnet, Hospital PNC, Unit PNC, Nursing Executive Leadership Council, Royal Oak Nursing Clinical Integration Council

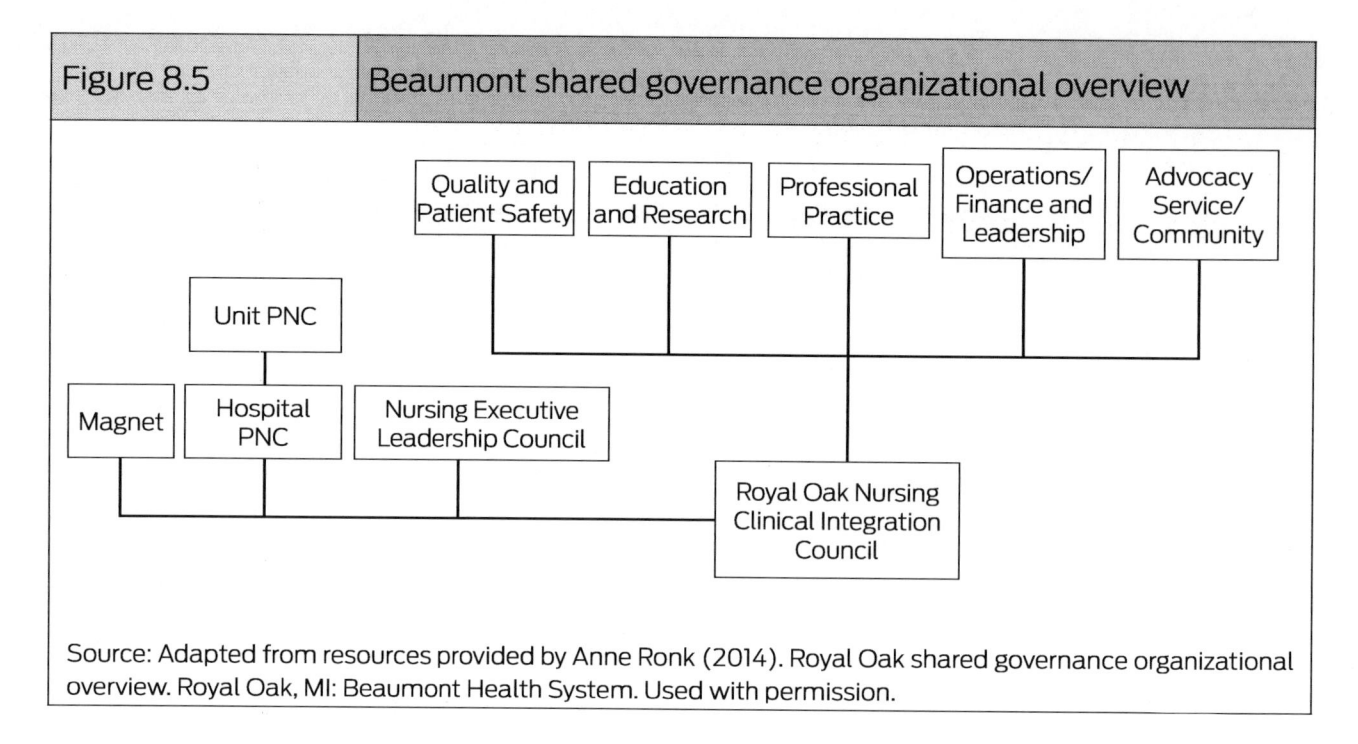

Source: Adapted from resources provided by Anne Ronk (2014). Royal Oak shared governance organizational overview. Royal Oak, MI: Beaumont Health System. Used with permission.

Shared governance in action

The formal rollout of the new nursing shared governance model shown in Figure 8.5 will not occur until fall 2014. However, a great example of shared governance in action has been the journey the PNC redesign team has been on for the past 18 months. This team was given the responsibility and support to completely change the nursing decision-making and leadership structures. The redesign team is composed of managers and staff nurses working collaboratively—no group more important than the other. This team is often asked for input into critical decisions by the CNO. It was used as a pilot for how the new structures might function. There is great excitement and eagerness for the new model and a true anticipation of the transformation of nursing shared governance at Royal Oak Beaumont Hospital.

Case Study 2

King Hussein Cancer Center (KHCC), Amman, Jordan

Contributing authors: Majeda A. Al-Ruzzieh, PhD(c), MSN, RN, Director of Nursing Services, Certificate Holder in Fundamentals of Magnet®, ANCC U.S., and Chairperson KHCC Steering Committee for Magnet®, and a member of the Executive Board for Jordanian Nursing Council; Mohammad Awwad, PhD, Nurse Manager for MRP program, KHCC

This example details the inner workings of shared governance in the King Hussein Cancer Center (KHCC) in Amman, Jordan. Consider how the process is similar as it unfolds despite the differences in culture and practice setting.

Effective nursing leadership is important in all nursing roles, whether the nurse practices in the field of education developing future leaders, as a researcher who mentors new researchers, as an administrator who provides support and guidance to staff, as a practitioner who provides exemplary care and shares professional knowledge, or as one who provides direction and support to practice through policy development.
—A. Squires

Background

KHCC was founded in 1997 as Al-Amal Cancer Center, which means "the center of hope" in Arabic. In 2002, there was an official ceremony to change the name of the center to honor the late King Hussein, who had died of cancer. KHCC is a comprehensive cancer center in Amman, Jordan, providing care to both adult and pediatric patients. The mission of KHCC is providing state-of-the art comprehensive cancer care to the citizens of Jordan and the region. Additionally, the mission is to provide access to education, training public awareness, and research in order to decrease mortality and alleviate suffering from cancer with the highest ethical standards and quality of care. KHCC was the first hospital in Jordan to be accredited by Joint Commission International Accreditation in 2006 and the first cancer center outside of the United States to receive Clinical Practice Certification Accreditation in cancer care.

Nursing services began with the establishment of KHCC in 2002. The focus then was on building nursing manpower and maximizing the capabilities of nurses by training and mentorship. Many professional and accreditation awards followed the late accreditation at hospital and departmental levels, ensuring care is provided according to the highest and most updated professional standards. For example, in 2013, Dr. Afeef Al-Ruzzieh, a genuinely transformational leader, won the HRH Princess Muna al-Hussein Award for Nursing Leadership and Management in Jordan (Rufaida Alaslamiah Medal), reflecting the transformational leadership at KHCC.

Additionally, Dr. Majeda Afeef Al-Ruzzieh, the director of nursing, is facilitating the journey to MRP designation with the help and support of Dr. Mohammad Awwad, the nurse manager for MRP, and her team. Dr. Afeef Al-Ruzzieh's roles include leading and managing all nursing services. She established shared governance for the nurses at KHCC and continues to monitor and evaluate all related structures and processes. Her commitment to shared governance is seen in such examples as:

- Establishing a dedicated unit for nursing research and EBP to support the professional nursing practice and development
- Becoming a member of the advisory board for the Shared Governance Forum
- Focusing her doctoral studies on transformational leadership and shared governance in nursing

In 2009, the nurses started their formal journey toward MRP excellence by implementing shared governance, establishing nursing research, and promoting evidence-based nursing practice at the unit level. Later, Dr. Mohammad Awwad became the nurse manager for the MRP program to continue moving the MRP forward. He provides oversight, coordination, and communication of all MRP-related activities at KHCC. Dr. Awwad worked as a nurse supervisor of research and EBP and serves as an institutional review board member at KHCC. He coordinates and arranges many nursing scientific activities in Jordan and has given many oral talks in nursing scientific meetings. He is a strong leader and actively engaged in advancing shared governance at KHCC.

Currently, the total number of beds at KHCC is 200, and that will be doubled in the new expansion by 2016 in order to meet the increased demands for cancer care in Jordan. Their journey toward developing a distinguished nursing organization began when the nursing department implemented shared governance as a management strategy and a core element in the Professional Practice Model for nurses (see Figure 8.6). The decision to implement shared governance resulted from a commitment to make KHCC a place where nurses practice with autonomy for better patient care and a supportive working environment.

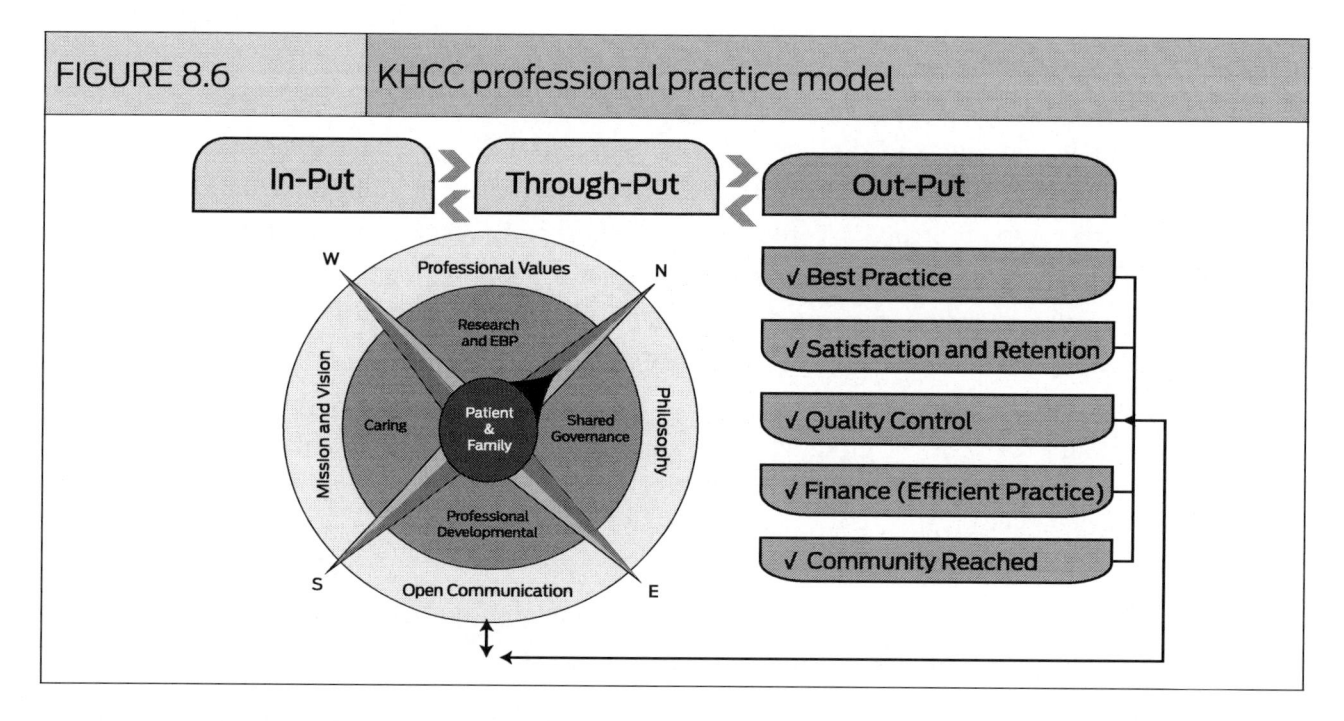

FIGURE 8.6 — KHCC professional practice model

Shared governance from inception

Shared governance started in 2010, when each nursing unit established a unit-based council (UBC) with 10%–20% of nurses' membership from total registered nurses. A model for UBC is guiding the council activities; the nurses in collaboration with the nurse managers developed this model (see Figure 8.7 for the KHCC model). In each UBC, the nurses discuss quality, practice, competency, and work environment topics in their units. The nurse managers were acting as mentors for nurses in the early stages of UBC development; both the nurses and the nurse managers received workshops and training to support them in their new roles. The unit-level council is responsible for:

- Encouraging communication, collaboration, innovation, and collegiality in all patient-care issues and working environments in the unit.
- Facilitating the continuous development and improvement in quality of care provided, competencies of the nurses, and excellence of practice in the unit.
- Supporting and encouraging mentorships for nurses at all levels.
- Building awareness about shared governance was continued throughout the process. For example, resources have been allocated by the general director, the director of nurses, and many supporters throughout KHCC, including library services, nursing education, human resources, and others.

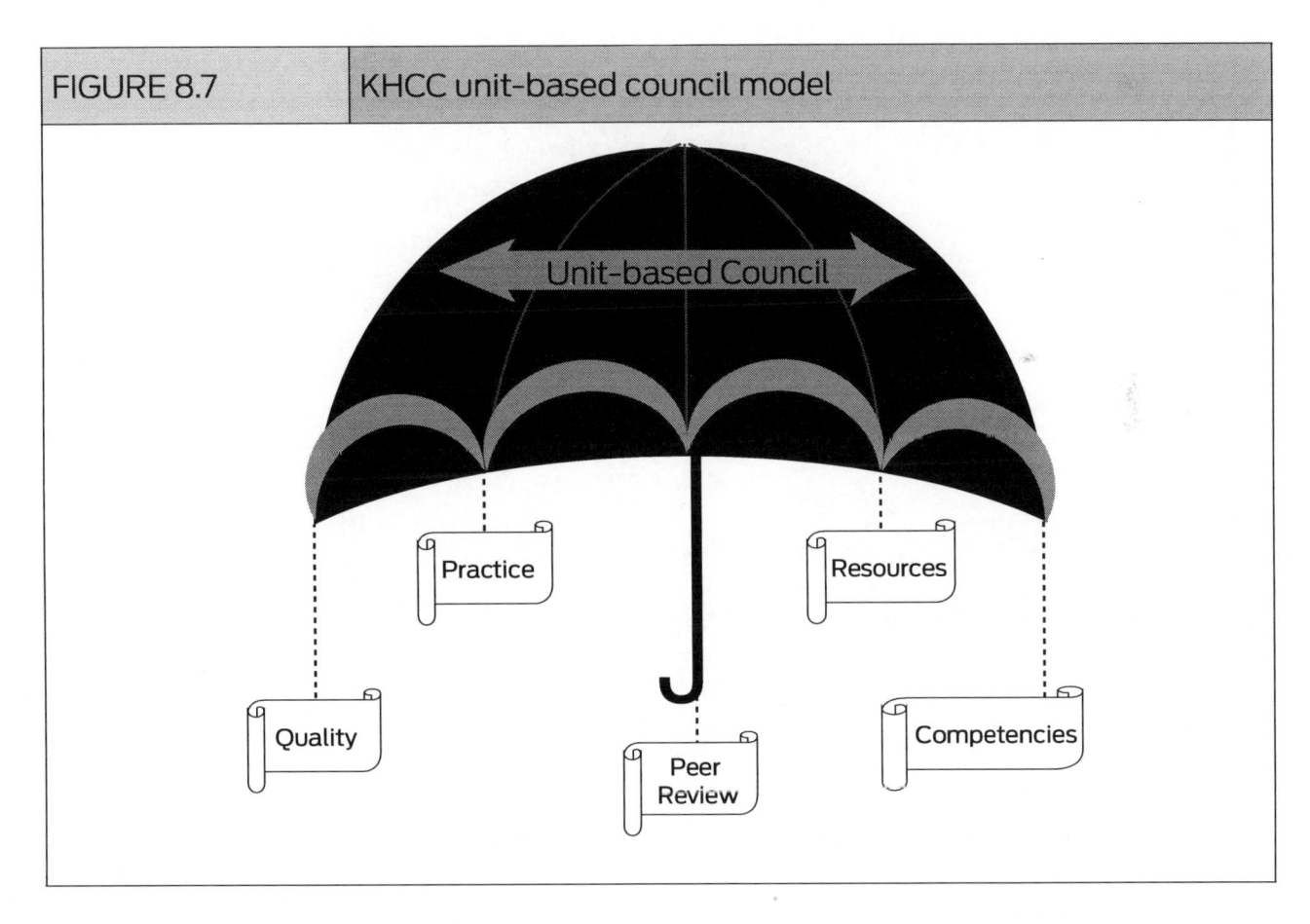

FIGURE 8.7   KHCC unit-based council model

[Umbrella diagram labeled "Unit-based Council" with scrolls: Quality, Practice, Peer Review, Resources, Competencies]

Implementation

In 2011, the shared governance structure expanded in order to have a bigger "umbrella" that coordinated and oversaw all activities of unit councils. A total of seven governance councils were formulated, which include practice, quality improvement, nursing research, evidence-based, nurse advocacy, leadership, professional development, and coordinating councils (see Figure 8.8 for the KHCC shared governance structure). Initially each council chair was a nurse manager who mentored the council cochair nurse (as successors) in order to lead the council independently later, an approach that supported the nurses who are young and with less nursing experience. At KHCC, the average age for the nurse is 25 years old, and the average experience is three years of nursing practice after graduation from nursing school.

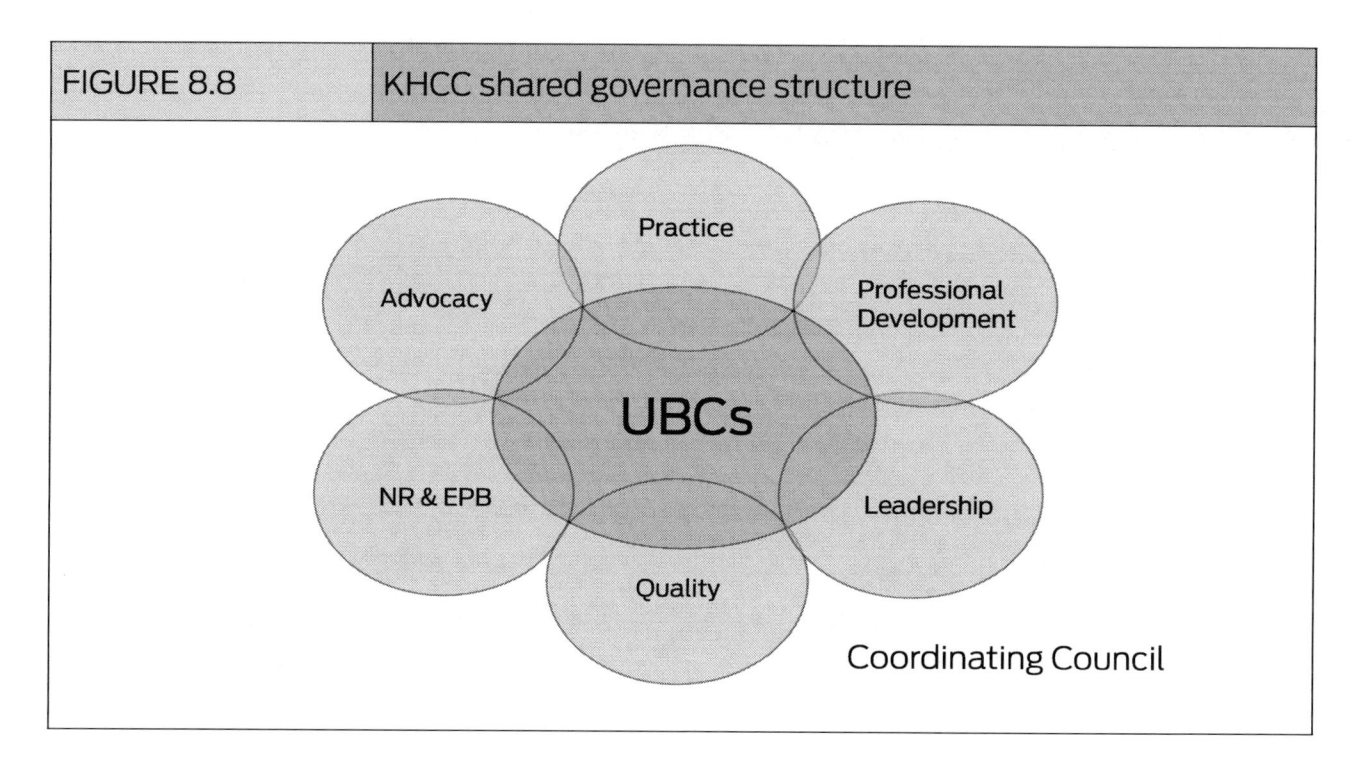

FIGURE 8.8   KHCC shared governance structure

A diagram showing overlapping circles labeled Practice, Advocacy, Professional Development, NR & EPB, Leadership, and Quality surrounding a central circle labeled UBCs, all within a Coordinating Council.

Original structure and responsibilities
Practice council

The council is responsible for maintaining the standards for clinical nursing practice:

- Review, revise, and approve policies and procedures and standards of care for nursing practice
- Integrate nursing research and evidence into nursing practice
- Integrate the professional practice model into aspects of care
- Develop and revise the care-delivery systems
- Implement peer review strategies

Quality improvement council

The council is responsible for the quality of nursing care and performance improvement:

- Coordinate the performance improvement and patient-safety activities with particular emphasis on systems improvement related to nursing practice and care outcomes
- Endorse and monitor department and unit-level quality improvement plans
- Review and evaluate the structure and outcomes quality indicators in comparison with benchmarking database
- Monitor registered nurses' satisfaction survey tools and results
- Collaborate with other disciplines in all quality-related matters

Professional development council

The council is responsible for nurses' professional development, including the following:

- Determine the educational and training needs for all nurses from all levels
- Facilitate nurses' professional development
- Foster the supportive environment for nursing professional advancement
- Assess and evaluate the nursing professional advancement program

Nursing advocacy council

The council is responsible for recognition and rewards for nurses:

- Create and maintain nursing recognition
- Support the positive working conditions for nurses
- Implement strategies that are supportive for a positive nursing image
- Promote the recruitment and retention of professional nurses

Research and EBP council

The council oversees research and EBP for nursing practice:

- Assist nursing in doing nursing research
- Assist nurses to use the published research and EBP for nursing practice
- Provide education and training for nurses related to research and EBP
- Facilitate partnership in research with universities and other institutions
- Monitor the model for EBP at KHCC

Leadership council

The council is responsible for overseeing all needs for nursing leadership development:

- Promote supportive environment for leadership development
- Evaluate the needs for training and advancement for all levels of nurse leaders at KHCC
- Integrate the EBP into leadership and management for nurses
- Discuss strategies to support and facilitate the nurses in other councils

Coordinating council

The council oversees all activities of the governance councils:

- Ensure closed-loop communication for all council activities
- Support and endorse all other council activities
- Approve and communicate all other council updates and decisions

Best practices to support shared governance

Participation and membership

At early stages of shared governance implementation, the nurse managers selected the nurses from their units to participate in shared governance councils and supported them. After one year, the councils were reformulated as per charters; nurses were selected the council to participate in according to their interests and qualifications. Practice and quality improvement councils include one RN from every nursing unit to ensure representation in those high-importance councils. Clinical nurses represent 70% of the total council members; some councils include non-nursing members in order to support their activities, such as a quality department representative in the quality council, and a human resources representative in the professional development council. At the staff level, the RNs are the only voting members in the UBC, also including the unit manager and educator as non-voting facilitators.

The research council includes non-nursing members to support its functions, which include: a librarian, a research officer, and two PhD faculty members from nursing schools. The addition of other colleagues and interprofessional partners provides access to resources, valuable experience, and mentorship for nursing research and EBP. Other councils invite a temporary non-voting member to be in the council upon their need. The renewal of membership for each member occurs annually, except for the chair and cochair who serve for two years. Upon renewal, every council will maintain 50% of old members in order to ensure smooth transition and to support the new members. All members receive orientation to their roles, the governance structures, and the communication between his or her unit and the council. Clear charters for the councils guide the members and the chairpersons in their roles.

Allocate time and resources

The key element for nurses' involvement is the leadership support in allocating time and resources for the nurses to facilitate their participation in the councils. The nurses' time to attend and perform the council work is paid time; four hours per month is compensated for meeting attendance and related council activities. The council chair can recommend extra time for the members in collaboration with the nurse managers if the council activities justify the increase. The general rule is to avoid meeting time during nurses' days off to maintain work-life balance and satisfaction.

Other resources were allocated according to the council needs and reflected in the department budget every year. An expanded electronic database for published research, new books, online courses, and classroom education are also provided. Additionally, standardized forms for council meeting minutes, charters, the model, and attendance sheets are provided to council chairs and explained to the members. Frequent monitoring for resource utilization is implemented to ensure the nurses have access to those resources.

Effective participation

During evaluation of the KHCC shared governance structure, there was an observed variation among councils in terms of effectiveness and achievement. The nursing leadership developed some strategies to handle ineffectiveness. The first strategy was to focus on education and increased awareness for members about their roles in the councils. This focus was reinforced by leaders' attendance at their council meetings to provide guidance and mentorship. Other strategies include development of evaluation tools to measure members and chairperson performance. The evaluation tool includes self and chairperson evaluation for a member and self and coordinating council evaluation for the chairperson. The evaluation will be done annually, and there will be consistent coaching throughout the year if needed. Each council will present a quarterly report to the coordinating council detailing council activities, challenges, and future plans. Monitoring and follow-up helps the members to prioritize the council mission and goals.

Closing the communication loop

A year after all the councils started, it became clear there was a lack of communication among the councils, and nurses reported that the changes in policies and procedures were not consistent. The difficulty in closing the loop led to creating new methods and tools. The coordinating council oversaw all plans and monitored the quarterly reports more closely. A communication form was created; the form indicated the topic under change and the proposed actions by the council. All communication forms will now be submitted to the facilitator of the coordinating council, who will forward the communication to the appropriate council and give written feedback to all communications. A logbook for all communication was created to monitor the implementation. The number of initiatives to improve care was obviously increased after implementing the communication form.

Developing leadership skills

Ensuring leadership competency for the councils' chairpersons was and remains the key element to succeed. A leadership course was conducted in order to support the councils' leaders. Each council has a cochair who will be mentored for his or her leadership skills as a future council leader. Additionally, the council has a leadership advisor who attends the meeting for mentoring without voting.

An evolving process

The shared governance model at KHCC has continued to evolve and mature. Each nursing unit developed a communication "tree" where each nurse has a cohort of four to five RNs to update on council activities and also to take their recommendations to the respective councils. Shared governance is part of the orientation for the new nurses, and its support is part of all job descriptions for nurses at KHCC. The current need is to reevaluate the professional practice model and define strategies for implementation and enculturation.

Nursing administration at KHCC supports shared governance, as patient outcomes improve after implementation at the unit level, and RNs' satisfaction improves by having a voice to change nursing practice and quality of care. The administrators have more focus on strategic planning and organizational initiatives. Both clinical nurses and managers are collaborating in decisions related to better care and supportive working environments. Although nurses are young and have less practice experience, they are enthusiastic—ready to learn and change for better opportunities. They are proud to be part of the first institution in Jordan implementing shared governance and to see the changes blossom.

Chapter 9

Relationships for Excellence

Advantages of ISO Quality Management and the ANCC Magnet Recognition Program®

> *Improved statistics would tell us more of the relative value of particular operations and modes of treatment than we have any means of ascertaining at present ... and the truth thus ascertained would enable us to save life and suffering, and to improve the treatment and management of the sick ...*
>
> *It need hardly be pointed out of what great practical value these and similar results would become ... hospitals might be compared with hospitals and wards with wards. The whole question of hospital economics as influenced by diets, medicines, comforts, could be brought under examination and discussion.*
> —Florence Nightingale, Notes on Hospitals, 1863

Shared governance integrates systems of administration, education, management, and quality improvement and responsibilities, authority, and accountabilities. It is a process for reengineering organizations, changing the basic structures, strategies, and outcomes. Risk awareness and quality link cost and value to the management of processes related to the reengineering and implementation of shared governance to achieve excellence.

Two examples of quality, safety, competency, and value demonstrated through shared governance are: the International Organization for Standardization (ISO) and the American Nurses Credentialing Center (ANCC)—among others (see Appendix B for a comprehensive bibliography). These organizations recognize the critical involvement of all healthcare providers, including interprofessional partners and multidisciplinary team members. Let's take a closer look and see what they each contribute to the establishment, implementation, and sustainment of a culture of shared governance.

Shared Governance and ISO Quality Management

Contributing author: Logan Asbury, DBA(c), MBA, BS, SSBB

> *Not having a common understanding of quality puts more pain into an organization than anything else I have ever known.*
> —Philip Crosby, Let's Talk Quality, *1989*

Over the past two decades, the military and U.S. Department of Veterans Affairs (VA) have expanded and reconceived the healthcare provider roles as part of restructuring services and systems to meet the growing needs of veterans. Seeking better ways to operate more efficiently and effectively, they recognized how critical providers are in reducing and preventing medical errors and infections, in establishing and maintaining quality of services and care, as well as transitioning patients from hospital to home, especially when providers lead these efforts in collaboration with interprofessional partners and multidisciplinary team members (Institute of Medicine [IOM], 2011; *http://www1.va.gov/health/*).

With so many agencies surveying and auditing performance and processes in healthcare organizations, there is a growing need for healthcare providers to gain a broader knowledge of national and international standards with applications to practice (e.g., accreditations and certifications from The Joint Commission, the National Database for Nursing Quality Indicators [NDNQI], the American Society for Quality [ASQ], and the ISO). The goal over the long term is to exceed customer and organizational expectations through a set of efficient, accountable, and measurable processes within the context of excellence in healthcare. To effect change and continual improvement, it is important to understand and implement process-based quality management systems.

What is ISO?
Since 1947, ISO has published more than 18,500 International Standards with roots in engineering, construction, agriculture, medical devices, information technology developments, and soon, healthcare services. ISO does not include requirements specific to other management systems (e.g., those particular to occupational health and safety management, environmental management, or risk management) but does enable an organization to align and integrate its own quality management system (QMS) with related management system requirements.

ISO is a non-governmental organization bridging public and private sectors. It has a global community of member bodies. ISO uses technical committees representing their sectors of expertise to prepare standards with international applications and use. Each member body votes to accept standards, which apply to organizations, people, products, and services of that nation.

Process-based quality management with ISO 9001:2008

Efficiency is doing things right;
effectiveness is doing the right things.
    —Peter Drucker

Organizations inside and outside of healthcare perform various activities to meet and exceed customer expectations. When a set of activities uses resources to transform inputs into outputs, it is considered a process. Organizations are composed of various interacting processes where the output of one process is often the input of another. These interacting processes focus around achieving organizational objectives and work together to form an integrated whole: the organization's system. ISO 9001:2008 serves as the blueprint for building an effective process-based quality management system and facilitates an environment for the efficient management of an organization's system of processes to provide:

- Consistent service,
- Increased customer satisfaction, and
- Continual improvement of the organization

ISO and the PDCA cycle

ISO 9001:2008 promotes the adoption of a process approach, the Shewhart Cycle, to create, implement, and improve an organization's QMS. The Shewhart Cycle, more commonly known as the "Plan-Do-Check-Act" (PDCA) cycle, is used to develop, implement, track, monitor, and improve all processes within the QMS. This approach allows an organization to gain control over its interrelated processes and grants them the ability to manage these processes as a system. Managing processes as a system allows an organization to effectively and efficiently achieve its objectives by meeting and exceeding customer requirements.

PDCA consists of four steps easily implemented at service, practice, and unit levels:

- **Plan:** Identify and establish goals, objectives, and processes needed to deliver the desired outcomes
- **Do:** Implement the process(es) developed and established by the service, practice, or unit
- **Check:** Monitor, measure, and evaluate the implemented processes by testing the results against the predetermined goals or objectives
- **Act:** Take actions necessary to continually improve process performance and service outcomes

The ISO standard is not prescriptive; organizations determine how they will meet their requirements. Though each QMS may be unique, organizations conforming to the ISO requirements are considered equals in terms of quality management (e.g., as with Joint Commission standards, ANCC Magnet® criteria for empirical outcomes, and Baldrige National Quality Program criteria).

What does ISO have to do with shared governance?

ISO is a quality management system of processes that recognizes 90%–95% of all defects are due to process failure, not people failure. Like those in shared governance structures, ISO process-based systems:

- Reduce the cost of poor performance and system redundancies
- Establish and streamline processes through documentation
- Identify weaker areas of the system for improvement
- Provide an environment for consistency and predictability of output to meet customer, regulatory, and stakeholder requirements
- Complement other management systems (e.g., Lean, Six Sigma)
- Provide effective and efficient control of processes by management, which includes:
    » Leading, directing, and controlling to achieve a specified outcome
    » A planned group of activities to be carried out
    » Coordination of activities and use of resources within the organization to meet specified goals
- Provide for self-evaluation by the organization, which includes:
    » Cost reduction (profit enhancer)
    » Continual improvement
    » Effective management control
- Clearly define roles, responsibilities, and information flow by process
- Support provider involvement and ownership of processes at points of service
- Validate competencies
- Increase stakeholder confidence (e.g., leaders, providers, patients, interprofessional and multidisciplinary team members, and others)

The most successfully designed and implemented management structures involve top management (i.e., leaders within the management system scope) and the people performing the tasks and activities, especially at points of service. ISO standards provide a foundation for the development of a management (governance) structure that facilitates movement from an environment of micromanagement and transactional leadership to one of shared governance and transformational leadership. Engagement with healthcare providers helps define the right amount of management control to ensure an effective and efficient quality system of shared decision-making at the points of service.

As people (e.g., direct-care providers, advanced practice nurses, physicians, pharmacists, social workers), technologies, environments of care, and customers (e.g., patient populations, communities of practice) change, quality management control systems must change, too. Measurement and review systems are needed to monitor and forecast changes and maintain the right amount of management control and shared leadership.

ISO standards form a quality and business management system that can provide organizations a process-based approach to managing daily operations and supporting relationships with stakeholders—patients, healthcare providers, and suppliers. ISO helps organizations define and guide the right amount of management control within the context of eight quality management principles for sustained performance improvements. These eight principles (with adaptations to healthcare and shared governance added) include:

1. **Customer focus:** Organizations depend on their customers and must understand current and future needs, striving to meet and exceed customer requirements and expectations (e.g., primary care, patient-centered care, medical home models, clinical nurse leaders, hospitalists)

2. **Leadership:** Establish purpose and direction of organization (i.e., service, practice, and unit); create and maintain internal environments in which providers can become fully involved in achieving the goals and objectives of the organization and the discipline or service:
   - Leadership begins with the mission (how organizations define the reasons for their existence) and identifies who the customer is (customer focus and leadership)
   - Top management communicates the mission and where they want to direct the organization (vision) to the employees to engage them in the process (leadership and involvement of people)

3. **Involvement of people:** Employees at all levels and points of service are the essence of the organization; their full involvement enables them to contribute to the organization (i.e., shared governance and engagement)

4. **Process approach:** A desired result or outcome is achieved more efficiently when activities and related resources are managed as a process (i.e., governance)
   - The organization can engage its people in defining the processes in support of the mission and vision (process approach, involvement of people, and leadership)
   - Connected processes form the management system designed to meet the organization's mission and vision (system approach to management, leadership, and customer focus)

5. **System approach to management:** Identifying, understanding, and managing interrelated processes as a system contributes to the organization's effectiveness and efficiency in achieving its objectives

6. **Continual improvement:** Improving the organization's overall performance should be a permanent goal and objective of the organization:
   - Once the management system is defined, the organization will have measurements and data needed to continually improve the effectiveness of its QMS (system approach to management, factual approach to decision-making, continual improvement, and customer focus)
   - These measurements can have significant impact on quality when direct-care providers participate at practice and unit levels through shared governance activities at points of service (e.g., central quality councils, practice and unit councils)

7. **Factual approach to decision-making:** Effective decisions are based on the analysis of data and information, evidenced in changes in practice to improve patient and employee safety and service outcomes

8. **Mutually beneficial supplier relationships:** An organization and its suppliers are interdependent and have a mutually beneficial relationship that enhances the ability of both to create value (e.g., surgical suppliers, administrative and clinical supplies, products, and services related to healthcare):
   - It is mutually beneficial to involve suppliers to help with the organization's customer focus (mutually beneficial supplier relationship and customer focus)
   - Examples of such relationships (mutually beneficial supplier relationship and customer focus) include:
     » When an equipment supplier provides training on how to safely and effectively use the equipment
     » When suppliers and customers share information and data to improve products and services

The purpose of quality management is to ensure products and services achieve customer satisfaction through customer-oriented processes. This is best achieved at points of service through engaged interprofessional and multidisciplinary team members. Practice- and unit-level councils provide a structure for identifying, monitoring, and evaluating quality of services and care to facilitate continual performance and process improvement in practice settings.

Senior leaders with managers and supervisors create a work environment that fully engages employees, one in which QMS can operate effectively, and in which leadership is demonstrated by:
- Following through with communication and task completion
- Providing direction and guidance

- Suppling tools and resources to be successful
- Practicing flexibility—ability to adopt, adapt, or abandon; to adjust plans wherever needed

NOTE: *The material in the paragraphs above describing ISO's relevance to shared governance was adapted from a presentation by ISO Consultants for Healthcare (ICH). (November 15–19, 2010). "ISO9001:2008 lead auditor for international quality management systems with applications for healthcare." Dayton, OH: ICH. For questions or more information, please contact: Ted Schmidt, Chris Kolb, or William J. Metzcar, Executive Oversight, Det Norske Veritas Surveyor, at wmetzcar@ich-global.com.*

Tying ISO to Shared Governance in Healthcare

Complexity creates confusion, simplicity focus.
—Edward de Bono

Shared governance provides a structure in which providers implement and maintain a process approach for managing quality to drive innovation and continual improvements in services and organizational stewardship (e.g., business practices and fiscal responsibilities) at points of service.

Presently, the use of ISO standards inside healthcare-delivery systems, facilities, and support networks is an open market. The QMS within ISO and shared governance are designed to incorporate standardization of processes and procedures, products, organizational structures, and execution of services. The intent is:

- Standardization with service-specific customization to streamline the workload
- To improve the effectiveness of the organization and the services it supports
- To enhance efficiency through shared decision-making and shared leadership

The use of ISO standards within a healthcare facility, setting, or scope of practice stands to realize cost savings while empowering employees, thereby increasing satisfaction. An example from military medicine is the standardization of the professional credentialing process of providers within all military treatment facilities and outside Department of Defense (DoD) entities. The system currently in place may be similar; however, duplication and redundancies are present in every military facility and branch of military service, as well as civilian-supported military entities. Military installations have become Joint Bases and operate in every realm of the DoD to include the Veteran's Affairs (VA) system with some interoperability. ISO, coupled with shared governance, offers healthcare providers an opportunity to streamline processes, reduce variances, and eliminate redundancies through shared decision-making around professional practice and credentialing.

Why ISO 9001:2008?

The ANCC established its accreditation program in 1974 to recognize organizations (or components of organizations) providing high-quality continuing education for nurses at all levels of practice. In 2007, ANCC received ISO 9001:2008 certification in all of its credentialing programs, including professional services rendered in the administration of the MRP for excellence in nursing in healthcare organizations, the accreditation program for excellence in continuing nursing education, Pathway to Excellence® Program for excellence in healthcare organizations, and the certification program.

ANCC recognized how organizations implementing an ISO 9001:2008 QMS achieved important benefits: a more organized operating environment, effective and efficient operations, improved employee morale, increased staff engagement, and improved customer satisfaction. Implementation of an ISO 9001 QMS helps to build a strong quality culture of ownership, accountability, and overall improved performance. Roles and responsibilities are clearly articulated, processes are defined and documented, and an overall culture of standardization, consistency, and quality results are realized through shared governance and professional autonomy. In achieving ISO certification, ANCC effectively demonstrated that all of its programs, products, and services are based on uniform policies and standards. (Adapted from the description of the ANCC ISO journey: *www.nursecredentialing.org/ FunctionalCategory/AboutANCC/ISOJourney.aspx.*)

Shared Governance and Magnet Recognition Program® (MRP)

Contributing author: Sylvia Brown, MSN

> *I find the important thing in life is not where we are,*
> *but in what direction we are moving.*
> —Oliver Wendell Holmes

The mission of the ANCC is to recognize healthcare organizations globally for nursing excellence, quality patient care, and innovations in nursing practice through credentialing programs and related services. One of these is the ANCC MRP, the "Nobel Prize" of nursing excellence in professional practice environments.

The relationship between shared governance and the MRP is a synergistic one. Shared governance is a process form of structure for autonomous direct-care nurses to come to the table and share their experiences and secure decision-making power in an organization. Shared governance asks, "What decision have you made lately?" Achieving MRP is a cultural, transformational journey. MRP and shared governance must be a part of the strategic plan for the organization when nursing excellence is the standard of professional practice (Haag-Heitman and George, 2010).

ANCC MRP goals

The MRP embraces three primary goals:

1. Promote quality of healthcare services in a safe environment that supports competent, autonomous professional nursing practice
2. Identify excellence in the delivery of nursing services to patients and residents
3. Provide a mechanism for the dissemination of research, evidence, and "best practices" in nursing services

The journey to MRP shares two central elements with the shared governance process model—cultural enhancements and structural enhancements, as follows:

- **Cultural enhancements.** The work environment is changed during this process, enabling and empowering nurses at points of service to improve and enhance patient outcomes. The MRP journey will not be successful without a culture of shared decision-making and shared leadership among professional nurses, interprofessional partnerships, and a multidisciplinary team (clinical and administrative) first being in place.
- **Structural enhancements.** A strategic plan is built around the autonomy of nurses sharing in decision-making and functioning in four primary professional roles: clinical practice, education, research, and administration. Shared governance provides a professional practice environment in which nurses can develop and mature in these roles to effectively enhance the organizational culture.

Benefits of the ANCC MRP and shared governance

Three groups reflect and build the five Components and 14 Forces of Magnetism® into their culture:

- Those who have implemented shared decision-making, professional nurse autonomy, and the essentials of the 14 Forces of Magnetism and are ready to articulate them
- Those who are putting the essentials in place and beginning to change the culture before demonstrating it through the application for MRP recognition
- Those who have chosen to implement the essentials of the culture but may not apply for formal consideration or designation by ANCC

The benefits of MRP for organizations include the ability to:

- Attract and retain top talent through increased staff satisfaction and retention, reduced employee burnout, and decreased vacancies and turnover
- Continually improve care, safety, and satisfaction
- Create and build an engaged, collegial, and collaborative culture through team-building, quality improvement, shared decision-making, and shared leadership activities

- Advance standards of practice and performance, research and evidence-based practice, and care-delivery systems
- Expand business and financial stability and growth

Shared governance helps those in leadership positions provide a professional practice environment that supports and facilitates healthcare provider and direct-care nurse autonomy in:

- Determining education and certification credentials
- Evaluating and writing research
- Writing and updating policies and procedures
- Participating in scheduling
- Managing their own competencies
- Providing in-services and continuing education
- Preceptoring students, new graduates, and new employees
- Any other duties they are interested in learning and participating in with their nurse management or leadership, interprofessional partners and multidisciplinary team members, and administration

These qualities and characteristics evident in MRP organizations have long been reflected in the effective shared governance processes and outcomes described by such researchers as Havens and Aiken (1999), Havens and Vasey (2003), Porter-O'Grady (1986, 1990, 1992, 2002, 2003c, 2004, 2008, 2009c, 2010a), and Hess (1994a, 1998a,b, 2013). See Appendix 37 for a collection of 2013 shared governance articles and research.

Essentials of service excellence

"Eight essentials of magnetism" are evident in every culture of shared governance. They indicate factors that keep nurses working in professional practice environments (McClure and Hinshaw, 2002). These same indicators influence all healthcare providers, interprofessional partners, and multidisciplinary team members engaged in shared decision-making and shared leadership.

1. **Working with clinically competent nurses:** Direct-care nurses participate in identifying their own competencies each year based on what's new, changed, problematic, and high-risk and time-sensitive in the practice environment; verify how they meet those competencies; and collaborate with nurse leaders to identify and verify what organizational competencies also need to be addressed

2. **Good nurse-physician relationships:** Creation of collaborative interprofessional partnerships with mutual trust and respect, collegiality, and shared accountability

3. **Support for education:** Promotion of advanced credentialing through facilitation and flexibility of work schedules and resources provided (e.g., bringing academic education onto the facility campus out of respect for the work-life balance needs)

4. **Adequate staffing:** Participation in staffing schedules, which encourages engagement, involvement, and shared decision-making by staff who are thinking beyond the unit level to the organization as a whole

5. **Concern for the patient is paramount:** Do what is needed for staff first (e.g., providing resources and ongoing training to maintain and enhance competencies) so they can focus all their energy, expertise, and experience on meeting the needs of the patients, the essence of staff-centered, patient-focused, relationship-based care and service

6. **Autonomy and accountability:** Improve communication and delegation by bringing together partnership, equity, responsibility, authority, ownership, and accountability in shared decision-making and shared leadership in professional practice environments

7. **Supportive managers and supervisors:** The manager or supervisor is the key retention person at points of service; this role is critical to effective outcomes related to shared decision-making and implementation of the shared governance process model at unit and organizational levels

8. **Control over practice and environment**: Shared decision-making leads to better patient outcomes and partnerships among patients, healthcare providers, and multidisciplinary team members

Shared governance pulls everything together and transforms professional practice to provide an environment of excellence that flows well through the Components and Forces of Magnetism®. Through ongoing research with a growing body of evidence and best practices, nurses and other healthcare providers demonstrate continual advances embedded in shared decision-making and shared leadership at points of service. They enjoy collegial management and staff partnerships, collaborative practice among all members of the interprofessional and multidisciplinary teams, and accountability-based ownership in issues related to practice, quality, and competence.

Five Components

If the MRP is the "Nobel Prize" of nursing, the five Components and 14 Forces of Magnetism comprise its core, and shared governance constitutes their expression in healthcare. The Components and Forces are categories of attributes or outcomes that exemplify nursing excellence evidenced by shared decision-making, partnership, equity, responsibility, accountability, authority, and ownership in professional practice.

The 14 Forces of Magnetism are folded into the five Components and are fundamental to determining excellence in the professional nursing practice environment. In 2008, eight domains were also added to describe the model components of magnetism: leadership, resource utilization and development, models that guide practice and performance, safe and ethical practice, autonomous practice, quality processes, research, and outcomes.

MRP is about the journey. The Forces are based on compelling original research (McClure and Hinshaw, 2002) and make it easier to engage leaders, managers and supervisors, and direct-care providers in the processes of shared governance and the MRP journey to nursing excellence—even if they are not going for MRP designation or redesignation. The components of MRP are all relative to shared governance.

Transformational leadership

(Domain: Leadership) This is leadership that moves the organization toward best practice, nursing excellence, and high-quality nursing care for patients.

Force 1. *Quality of nursing leadership:* The chief nursing officer (CNO) is a knowledgeable and strong risk taker who provides a professional practice environment and philosophy for mutual advocacy and shared decision-making within nursing service among all direct-care nurses and nurse leaders. The CNO sits at the highest level of decision-making in the organization—at the senior leadership table—so all nurses' voices can be heard and their interests represented throughout the organization. The CNO, the ambassador for nursing service, protects nursing leaders and direct-care nurses from political and economic influences that could negatively impact patient-care outcomes and professional practice environments.

Force 3. *Management style:* The CNO and nurse leaders (e.g., managers, directors, supervisors, charge nurses) help direct-care nurses create vision, philosophy, and shared purpose through supportive discussion and reflective practice. Feedback is valued and communicated at all levels of the organization. Direct-care nurse leaders are visible, accessible, and committed to working closely with the multidisciplinary team and other direct-care providers. Nurse leaders provide support, encouragement, resources, boundaries, and protection through the shared governance organizational process model in matters of professional practice, quality, and competence. They foster a collaborative culture. Management styles are grounded in transformational, servant leadership and shared decisional processes with outcomes of shared leadership.

Structural empowerment

(Domains: Resource utilization and development) This speaks to a cultural environment where shared governance thrives.

Force 2. *Organizational structure:* The macrosystem has decentralized, flat organizational structures, creating a sense of partnership, equity, accountability, and ownership within professional practice environments. Typically, the CNO reports directly to a CEO and serves at the executive level of the organization. MRP has no criteria for how the organizational structure should look. However, there must be a structure and process of some kind in place that is dynamic and responsive to change. A formal structure is critical to manage employee involvement through a representative model. Every organization develops its models and cultures differently but includes strategic planning, shared decision-making, and staff responsiveness. The organization demonstrates strong nursing representation in council and committee structures and through a functioning and productive system of shared decisional processes. Shared governance is demonstrated within the organizational structure.

Force 4. *Personnel policies and programs:* Direct-care nurses are involved in decision-making about budgets, schedules, salaries, competencies, resources, and practice. They should be familiar with budgets and their roles and responsibilities related to organizational, practice, and unit stewardship. Salaries and benefits are competitive with community standards with opportunities for advancement and promotions, awards, and bonuses for exceptional services. Job descriptions, written by nurses in partnership with representatives from human resources, reflect the characteristics of the essentials of service excellence grounded in the tenets and scopes of professional nursing practice (e.g., direct-care nurses, clinical nurse leaders, clinical nurse educators, nurse managers, and advanced practice nurses). Organizations demonstrate commitment to their nursing staff and foster a shared governance environment to attract and retain top talent and advance nursing standards and practice through personnel policies and programs. The nursing staff provides quality patient care, nursing excellence, and innovations in professional nursing practice as they feel valued and respected by the organization.

> **A best practice in participative scheduling**
>
> Creative and flexible staffing models and schedules accommodate the many demands direct-care providers experience on their time and attention at work and at home. Increased patient acuities and workloads require negotiation and shared decision-making at points of service to maximize staff satisfaction. One innovative group of nurses worked with their manager to restructure their shift hours. The unit council studied the possibilities, conferred with other staff and nurses regarding the proposed changes in shift rotations, and successfully demonstrated how improved patient-care outcomes could positively support their proposal. After further negotiation with leadership and human resources, the unit council informed staff they could pilot a change in their 12-hour shift rotations to 3 a.m. to 3 p.m. and 3 p.m. to 3 a.m. for six months. The new schedule resulted in a more enthusiastic and engaged staff, fewer call-ins, realized improvements in patient satisfaction and care outcomes, and a deeper respect for nursing leadership and the process of shared decision-making.
>
> **Source:** Unit council members at the James A. Haley VA Healthcare System, 2009

Force 10. *Community and the healthcare organization:* Healthcare providers build relationships within and among all types of healthcare and community organizations. They develop strong partnerships supportive of positive patient outcomes and the health of the communities they serve through community collaboration, positive outcomes from collaborations, and allocating and using appropriate resources. Nurses in shared governance recognize and embrace their responsibilities to support community outreach activities resulting in their service and the organization being seen as strong, positive, and productive community citizens.

Force 12. *Image of nursing:* Environments promoting MRP and shared governance build and expand the image of nursing within the organization and community. Nursing service's contributions are recognized and rewarded. Other members of the healthcare team characterize nursing services as essential to the organization and integral to the overall well-being of patients. The direct-care nurse's voice is heard and respected in the governing or central councils, in other departments and divisions, and in their nurse-physician and multidisciplinary team member relationships, effectively influencing systemwide processes.

A best practice in building influence and the image of nurses

Contributing author: Sandra F. Law, MSN, Bay Pines, Florida

Nursing education set up basic professional portfolios with template dividers and distributed one to every certified nurse in the organization during Nurses' Week. Photographs of each certified nurse were taken and put on a colorful PowerPoint® slide, complete with his or her credentials, title, and the specialty or specialties of certification. All of the pictures were printed and became the cover for each nurse's portfolio. They were then folded into a looped program and shown during a formal recognition ceremony held during Nurses' Week. The CEO, the chief of staff, the CNO, nurse leaders, and other service leaders, with many of the nursing staff and their friends and colleagues, attended the ceremony. Each certified nurse was presented his or her portfolio by the CNO and had his or her picture taken with the leadership. Throughout this incredible program honoring the significant accomplishments of these exceptional nurses, the PowerPoint® loop with each and every one of their pictures and accomplishments played in the background. Afterward, one nurse brought his portfolio to the registration table and, with tears in his eyes, thanked those present for the "best Nurses' Week gift I have ever gotten!"

Force 14. *Professional development:* Successful nursing partnership, equity, accountability, and ownership in practice demand lifelong learning. A variety of structures, programs, and activities directed at developing and empowering employees are needed to help staff accomplish service and organizational goals, and achieve desired outcomes through professional development. Examples include:

- Quality orientations
- Career development services
- Academic and formal education
- Continuing education
- In-services
- Competency-based clinical, leadership, and management development

- Career development
- Professional certification
- Continuous learning environments
- Sufficient human and fiscal resources for professional development
- Excellence in clinical practice and leadership supported
- Advance practice and certification promoted
- Professional relationships, preceptors, and mentors established, built, and sustained

Exemplary professional practice

(Domains: Models that guide practice, safe and ethical practice, autonomous practice, and quality processes) This is demonstrated through shared governance by a nursing staff that practices autonomy, uses professional theory models in provision of care, and advances nursing standards and practice.

Force 5. *Professional models of care:* There is an important difference between professional practice models of care and care-delivery systems. Professional models of care are the basis of the discipline of nursing and consider which nursing theorists are used in the organization (e.g., Benner, Neuman, King, or Orem). These models provide a theoretical foundation on which to build research for contrasts and comparisons. Because no one theory covers all patient populations with their unique needs, organizations usually have several theories folded into their conceptual framework, theories that reflect the values and philosophies of each nursing service.

MRP defines a professional practice model as "the driving force of nursing care" (*The Magnet Model Components and Sources of Evidence: Magnet Recognition Program®*, 2008, p. 44). Shared governance practice councils delineate the models of care and make sure there is evidence hardwired into the organization. Shared governance also ensures that nurses have adequate resources to accomplish desired patient-care outcomes.

A *care-delivery system* is defined as "a system for the provision of care that delineates the nurses' authority and accountability for clinical decision-making and outcomes" (*The Magnet Model Components and Sources of Evidence: Magnet Recognition Program®*, 2008, p. 38). For example, team nursing is a care-delivery system. It is not a conceptual model of care. Rocchiccioli and Tilbury (1998) describe eight care-delivery systems still evident today: functional nursing, team nursing, primary nursing, primary-team nursing, total patient care, modular nursing, differentiated practice, and case management.

Nurses are accountable for their own professional practice models and the systems of care delivery selected for nursing service. Shared governance provides a process structure for assessments, strategic change, and ongoing evaluation of patient outcomes and care-delivery systems that promote professionalism, accountability, evidence-based practice, adaptation to regulatory needs, and a staffing system reflective of patient needs. Models of nursing care (e.g., the relationship-based care model) give nurses the responsibility, authority, and accountability necessary to provide and coordinate patient care at points of service (Wright, 2002). Nurses need to know they are all practicing under the same standards.

Force 8. *Consultation and resources:* Catalog local and national speakers brought in for training, nursing grand rounds, clinical nurse specialists (in consultative roles), experts and expertise available within the organization or made available by bringing in consultants, and taking field trips to other facilities to review and learn about best practices in nursing. The organization and nursing service provide adequate resources, support, and opportunities for these activities.

Force 9. *Autonomy:* This is a fundamental principle of shared governance: Direct-care nurses within the organization govern their own practice and share in making decisions affecting practice, quality, and competence. They partner with other healthcare providers and patients to deliver care at all points of service. Leaders facilitate nurses' success by providing the resources, support, encouragement, and boundaries they need to dispense patient-focused care. Transitions to shared governance can be very difficult for leaders, managers and supervisors, and healthcare providers. It can be difficult to facilitate autonomous practice, to give over duties and responsibilities believed to be owned by management or leadership. However, giving that shared authority and decisional power to staff is critical to a mature shared governance process, a changed culture, and implementation of the principles of shared governance and Magnet®.

Force 11. *Nurses are teachers:* Nurses can be collaboratively coordinated into community resources. Healthcare providers are in key positions to educate their patients and their communities in preventive healthcare practices. They have emergency preparation skills, healthcare and wellness knowledge, and safety skills through training and experience. These skills are highly attractive commodities in local communities, and can be collaborative opportunities.

> ### A best practice in community outreach
>
> **Contributing author: Paul F. Sink, Jr., Tampa, Florida**
>
> Paul F. Sink, Jr., a retired nursing education coordinator for a Community Living Center in Florida, coordinated the continuing nursing education provided for annual workshops on hurricane awareness for Tampa and surrounding communities. As part of a multidisciplinary team of healthcare providers, safety specialists, and subject matter experts, he worked to help the citizens remain safe, calm, and ready during the many hurricanes and tropical storms they struggled to endure each hurricane season, whether storms came or only threatened.
>
> Nurses educate, precept, coach, orient, and mentor other nurses, students, and patients within the organization. They get involved in the lifelong learning of others, both inside and outside their communities. Students from a variety of clinical and academic programs are welcomed, supported, and engaged. Affiliation agreements and contractual arrangements are mutually beneficial. In a shared governance practice setting, nurses are supported by leadership and expected to serve as educators and teachers to ensure a foundation for quality care, safety, and ongoing competencies. Nurse development and mentoring programs prepare preceptors to work with all levels of students.

Force 13. *Interdisciplinary relationships:* Shared governance creates a forum for direct-care nurses, interprofessional partners, and multidisciplinary team members to develop and enhance mutual respect, knowledge, competence, and a platform for essential and meaningful contributions toward quality clinical outcomes. Collaborative working relationships within and among the disciplines are actively cultivated and valued (Swihart, 2011; Porter-O'Grady, 2009c; Edmonstone, 2003).

New knowledge, innovations, and improvements

(Domain: Research) New knowledge and innovations are utilized within a shared governance structure to make improvements as identified and promoted to enhance patient care and outcomes.

Force 7. *Quality improvement (QI):* This is the process that advances continual improvement, consistency, customer service, and the quality of care and services within organizations, services, disciplines, departments, and units. It focuses on operational effectiveness, clinical processes, and outcomes. Evidence-based care, nursing excellence, and innovations in professional nursing practice are all driven by quality improvement and research.

> **Best practices of QI: Nursing case study investigations (CSI) in shared governance**
>
> **Contributing author: Michelle Jans, MSN, RN-BC, Bay Pines, Florida**
>
> The nursing CSI is a process for analyzing events around patient outcomes that resulted in either near misses or medical errors of varying degrees in practice settings. Each month, quarterly, or as needed, case studies are developed by direct-care nurses around real incidents identified through root cause analyses or incident reports, or tagged by nursing leadership and nurses as potential learning opportunities to improve patient outcomes. Nurses from all shifts, inpatient units, and practice settings identify clues to the underlying problem(s) that may have changed the outcome if recognized earlier. Using a detective-like method of inquiry, nurses are able to uncover critical and often-missed clues to help them see the bigger picture and solve the case to complete the following:
>
> - Diagnose learning needs
> - Implement advanced assessment skills, critical thinking, and evidence-based practice
> - Discover limited and incomplete data within policies that would help provide a more appropriate clinical pathway to the presenting clinical picture
> - Increase communication and collaboration among multidisciplinary team members
> - Improve documentation in content and context
> - Enhance professional practice skills (organization, prioritization, delegation, problem solving)
> - Engage in open and honest peer review
>
> Through shared exploration and problem solving, the nursing CSI has become an integral forum for nurses to achieve a greater level of excellence by way of careful consideration of the evidence in practice, evaluation of the clues along the way, and successful solutions to the case at hand.

Empirical outcomes

(Domain: Outcomes) An alignment of MRP and shared governance enhances patient outcomes within the context of high-quality nursing practices.

Force 6. *Quality of care:* It's about processes, structures, and outcomes. Quality of care explores the effectiveness of the system to support nursing and patient care. Nurses engaged in shared governance make meaningful decisions about quality practice at points of service. They are responsible for providing evidence-based care grounded in research that facilitates improved patient-care outcomes in quality-of-care decisions related to practice, quality, and competence.

Empirical quality outcomes are best realized in environments of care with shared governance. Quality and performance improvement are process-driven approaches, usually with specific steps for design, development, production, or service, and evaluation with validation and verification (e.g., performance measures) to guide definitions and achieve or exceed identified goals.

Nurses participate in quality practice at all points of service through shared governance at micro-, meso-, and macrosystem levels. The ISO and the ANCC—among others (see Appendix B for bibliographic resources)—recognize the critical involvement of all healthcare providers, including interprofessional partners and multidisciplinary team members, in establishing, implementing, and sustaining a culture of shared governance.

Chapter 10

Tips for Success

Lessons Learned and Best Practices

Shared by healthcare leaders, direct-care providers,
team leaders and other organizations and communities of practice

> *"Come to the edge," he said.*
> *They said, "We are afraid."*
> *"Come to the edge," he said. They came.*
> *He pushed them ... and they flew.*
> —Guillaume Appollinaire

We wrote this book to take some of the guesswork out of the various structures and processes behind shared governance and to provide some basic tools for establishing and developing shared governance at the practice, unit, and governance council levels. Throughout the preceding chapters and sections, a number of strategies, case studies, lessons learned, and best practices have been provided to make the daily operations of shared governance meaningful and successful.

In this chapter you will find a brief listing of additional tips and ideas to further enhance the shared governance process and your journey in transforming professional practice for today and tomorrow. The future of healthcare in organizations and emerging global communities of practice depends on where you go from here.

1. Schedule a daylong retreat away from the organization to prepare organizational and service leaders to implement shared governance. Discuss the role shared governance plays in the Magnet Recognition Program® (MRP) journey, if the organization plans to pursue MRP designation or redesignation. Have subject matter experts present topic discussions on specific points: leadership, shared governance partners, steering group formation, design team for the shared governance model, a business case for shared governance, roles and responsibilities of direct-care providers, interprofessional partners, and the multidisciplinary team members.

2. Create expectations for staff contributions, beginning with onboarding, extending into the new employee orientation, and continuing throughout their careers.

3. Have a town hall meeting at least once per quarter to facilitate open communication among interprofessional providers and staff, service and administrative leaders, and multidisciplinary team members. (Communicate, communicate, communicate!)

4. Administer the Index of Professional Nursing Governance (IPNG) and Index of Professional Governance (IPG) surveys to see how your organization measures up—help build the repository of information on the efficacy and value of shared governance in healthcare settings.

5. Visit Online Journal of Issues in Nursing to view articles like "XYZ" and "Shared governance: Is it a model for nurses to gain control over their practice?" at *www.nursingworld.org*.

6. Use journal clubs, for example, to bring research to the bedside and engage direct-care providers in evidence-based practice for developing and implementing advanced decision-making and critical thinking (see Appendix 24, a guide for enhancing practice through journal clubs).

7. Encourage direct-care providers to meet each year to review organizational competencies and practice and unit needs; determine which competencies they will focus on for that year (high-risk and time-sensitive, changed, problematic, and/or new). See Appendix 5, Wright's competency decision worksheet.

8. Train *every registered nurse* in each unit and practice setting to be charge or lead nurse. Rotate the role and responsibilities to encourage leadership skills development and shared decision-making among all team members.

9. Involve all staff members in preparing and adapting their schedules to accommodate the needs of their work area. Open staffing to flexible schedules and peer-negotiated days off. Leadership, managers and supervisors, should only step in if there are irreconcilable differences or stalemates, or to help employees with the process. Responsibility here, as in other areas of shared governance, must be coupled with appropriate levels of authority and accountability to be successful.

10. Communicate the process, expectations, roles, and responsibilities for employees engaged in shared decision-making throughout the organization, not just in units and practice areas.

11. Explore and validate management and leadership styles in the shared governance process model selected.

12. Make sure all executives, directors, supervisors, and managers are trained and engaged in the shared governance process model development before bringing staff into the mix. Otherwise, the service leaders may become confused or uncomfortable and sabotage the work before it even begins.

13. Recognize and celebrate those direct-care providers who represent their peers and patients on the shared governance councils and in the community. Support them through creative staffing, surprise celebrations, quiet encouragements, and provision of whatever resources they need to be successful.

14. Prepare, support, and encourage service and unit or practice change champions to help lead strategic change and facilitate the implementation of shared governance.

15. Display unit and practice exhibits, bulletin boards, and other learning events, staff activities, and staff celebrations and awards.

16. Create an organizational "who's who" of your best practice employees, change champions, and hospital heroes to share with the organization and community.

17. Celebrate every milestone and moment of excellence completed along the way to organizational change through shared governance.

18. Attend workshops and seminars on shared governance and leadership in professional practice.

19. Network with organizations that have implemented shared governance successfully or are just beginning their journey (several have been referenced in this book). Share best practices with them.

    - Networking example: Lessons learned from shared governance visits to U.S. hospitals from Laura Hailes, 2012 Roosevelt Scholar, University of Nottingham, United Kingdom (her story is published online at *www.sharedgovernance.org/*).

20. Incorporate *succession planning* into your organization—it is the key for every role within the shared governance structure, from unit practice council members to the chief nursing officer. Poor succession planning and employing a candidate who didn't fully support shared governance leads to embedding and sustainability issues.

21. Enlist your organization's support in the form of funding to cover frontline staff while they attend meetings. (Historically, this was often the first budget to be cut, creating a false sense of economy, as improvements in patient care were stilted or worse still, ceased. This had great implications across the organization. Giving staff a voice, then taking it away, leads to a decline in job satisfaction, staff retention, and patient outcomes.)

22. Encourage the use of ward managers, and recognize that this role requires a lot of training and education. The role of ward manager in a shared governance structure is more facilitative than controlling—a significant cultural shift from typical hierarchical management styles. Organizations that didn't invest time and resources in supporting their managers with this change will be faced major problems with implementation, embedding, and sustainability.

23. Once shared governance is fully implemented and the organizational culture is ready, begin the MRP, Pathway, Baldridge, or other journeys to excellence.

24. Share success stories peer-to-peer, unit-to-unit, practice-to-practice, staff-to-leaders, and leaders-to-staff. Select one each month to present at town hall meetings, at leadership meetings, during in-services, in cafeterias, and in elevators. Shared governance takes on a life of its own when it becomes real and exciting to those participating in it, generating creative and innovative ideas, encouragement, and enthusiasm from one another's experiences.

25. Use unit and practice councils to identify what is needed for direct-care employees to be successful in their own microsystems, for example:

    - Engaged managers and direct supervisors
    - Knowledge and mentoring for staff and managers in the principles, characteristics, and tools of shared governance
    - A commitment from the organization, from all services, and specifically from all members at unit practice levels that shared governance is the organizational management structure for how employees "do business" every day

26. Prepare, educate, and support managers and supervisors about the implications affecting staff ownership and management support. For many, this is a new way of managing their employees. Precept and mentor them in their roles, responsibilities, and accountabilities in shared decisional processes (see Appendix 4, council shared decision-making tool).

27. This is key: Make it clear that participating in a shared governance organizational management infrastructure and professional practice model is not optional. Ownership, engagement, and active participation in the professional communities of practice are *essential* and must not be by invitation. If participation in shared governance is optional, the option eventually becomes the rule. Incorporate shared governance participation into job descriptions, performance appraisals and evaluations, competencies, and peer review.

28. Take the time necessary to build an effective, efficient, safe infrastructure that supports sustainable behaviors related to ownership, autonomous practice, and shared decision-making at the practice or unit level and beyond.

29. Engage providers as practice and unit educators in shared governance. These educators are generally direct-care providers who are responsible for assessing, planning, coordinating, and evaluating the educational needs of the employees in their practices or units. They work closely with practice or unit council members, staff, and the manager or supervisor to identify educational programs and activities to develop and maintain staff competencies. These educators help staff provide quality care for the unique patient populations on their assigned units by facilitating a continuous learning environment. Other activities may include the following:

    - Identify in-service needs of staff with assistance and support of other clinicians.
    - Coordinate in-services with direct-care providers, interprofessional partners, multidisciplinary team members, and others.

- Schedule speakers for varied in-services based on assessed needs.
- Network with other practice and unit educators to share information and provide cross-training when appropriate.
- Publicize centralized staff education and learning activities.
- Maintain accurate records of individual staff members' attendance at in-services, programs, mandatory reviews, and external learning events.
- Enter training data into the organization's education tracking system.
- Help the staff retrieve the data whenever needed.
- Each month, practice and unit educators might attend meetings to discuss their roles and responsibilities and how their work fits into the overarching strategic plan for continuing education and staff development within the whole organization. They hold a great deal of respect, autonomy, and mutual accountability with the staff because they are helping ensure excellence in practice at all points of service.

30. Remember to look at the big picture:
    - Think long-te[rm] [...] actions; pay very close attention to the de[...]
    - Participate in [...] [orga]nization) level to better plan and engage a[...] [li]ne, division, or department) and microsy[...] sample health system model.
    - Alignment o[...] e is critical to the success of all three system[...]

[Sticky note: Shared Governance / Cost / A-3 / Visioning / Innovation Event / →Standards - templates, etc]

31. Never forget the [...] [mov]es us quickly beyond the practical to the p[...] [thr]eshold of a patient and family's door, he or she c[...] [pra]ctical preparation into that of a personal healing [...] [do]es is in service to the patient. This border cros[...] nd family's world—a world about which they know little—and within which they must tread with great humility."

32. Learn how to *fail forward* and turn mistakes and missteps into building blocks (Maxwell, 2007). Frequently reenergize staff and shared governance champions by looking at what is happening—not as a failure but as a point of stepping back to renew and refine some structures and processes—to build a stronger framework for the development of meaningful and sustainable professional practice within a shared governance model which exemplifies it.

33. Think *proactively*, not reactively. Stop and take a deep breath before moving forward, speaking, or acting. Ask questions. Step back and look at the situation or event from a new perspective. This is how a transformational leader approaches problems, crises, and other disasters, both potential and real.

34. Follow the advice of the Container Store's Elizabeth Barrett regarding human resources: Entrust your direct care providers with the responsibility for attracting, motivating, and retaining the best staff possible.

35. Create, maintain, and share professional portfolios. Follow one another's professional activities: presentations, academic advancements, certifications, and contributions through professional organizations, affiliations, committees, advisory boards, and other accomplishments. Encourage and support one another through shared possibilities and opportunities.

36. Solicit and apply best practices from other people, practices, units, disciplines, departments, and organizations.

37. Volunteer with enthusiasm! Take action!

38. Identify a practice or unit council facilitator to coordinate council activities:
    - Work closely with the manager or supervisor and direct-care providers to determine what activities, projects, and tasks are workable for change, development, or implementation
    - Identify practice and unit issues and concerns to bring before the council
    - Communicate issues, concerns, and outcomes to all direct-care providers and staff on all shifts through multiple approaches and venues

39. Create quarterly reports of activities, accomplishments, outcomes, and celebrations to record and communicate progress in improving and advancing professional practice, quality, and competency through shared governance and influencing decisions across the organization.

40. Take classes and courses not directly job-related (e.g., crucial conversations, how to do stand-up comedy, writing for everyone, blogging for exercise, and so on) to relax and energize creative thinking—and to provide more interesting icebreakers for practice and unit council meetings.

41. Collect and share professional journals, newsletters, and magazines in a break room, as a lending library, or in a cart. Consider setting up a resource for sharing URLs of interesting articles. Follow the advice of Scott Adams, who said "Share knowledge freely and ask others to do the same, ideally in small digestible chunks."

42. Make *teaching* a part of everyone's job description. Reward those who do a good job of communicating useful information to staff on all shifts, including off-tours (Adams, 1996).

43. Listen *actively* (invest in what is being said) to learn from others and adapt to include their perspectives. Teams need active listening to consider any issue or point of discussion from all sides and make clear and accurate decisions together.

44. Remember that everyone's job is important. Engage each person at the practice- and unit-level and beyond in the mission, values, and goals of the organization and each practice setting. Celebrate every contribution—large and small—to the safety and care of patients and their families.

45. Learn from students' and new employees' experiences and skills. Bring them into the practice or unit council as soon as possible. Do not lose the opportunities they bring to the table. New staff usually has a wealth of information, questions, and perspectives that can advance practice in interesting ways.

46. Be open and available to one another.

47. When participating in peer review, give feedback all along the way. Identify both positive accomplishments and opportunities to improve and grow as they occur and share them then. There should be no surprises at evaluation time.

48. Let people make mistakes—as long as they do not jeopardize staff or patient safety. This is an excellent way to impact learning and influence change.

49. Take 5 to 10 minutes before each practice or unit council meeting to receive information, questions, ideas, requests, and cautions from managers and supervisors. Sometimes, a practice or unit council agenda will change with new information. Then take 5 or 10 minutes at the end of each practice or unit council meeting to review what was learned, answer questions, and set goals for the next meeting.

50. Build on previously gained knowledge, experiences, and wisdom.

51. Set clear goals with time for feedback in both directions.

52. Avoid more predictable pitfalls possible when implementing shared governance:
    - Burnout by council members, staff members (e.g., those covering for staff representatives to attend central council meetings or to engage in assigned activities)
    - Decisions made in isolation (e.g., by one practice, unit, or council without engaging other employees or councils)
    - Repetitive or redundant work
    - Lack of employee engagement (e.g., service leaders, direct-care providers)
    - Discomfort by staff representatives when interacting with central councils and other staff members (e.g., feeling overwhelmed or unprepared)
    - Practice or unit council meetings become "just another staff—or management—meeting" with information-sharing but no actively shared decision-making or shared leadership evident

- Resistance or unintended sabotage by managers, supervisors, providers, or employees not participating or engaged in change or shared governance implementation at practice or unit levels
- Lack of knowledge, ability, or support to effectively engage in shared governance meetings and activities
- Poor or inconsistent structure of councils

53. Remember, everyone has a contribution to make. So what are *your* ideas for successful shared governance?

Chapter 11
The Forum for Shared Governance
International Clearinghouse for Research and Resources

Contributing author: Robert G. Hess, Jr., founder of the Forum for Shared Governance

In every art, beginners must start with models of those who have practiced
the same art before them. And it is not only a matter of looking ... it is a matter
of being drawn into the individual work of art, of realizing that it has been made
by a real human being, and trying to discover the secret of its creation.
   —Ruth Whitman

Founding the Forum

Despite 35 years of history, shared governance often remains difficult to implement. In 2005, I created the Forum for Shared Governance as a nonprofit clearinghouse for promoting and disseminating research about shared governance and similar organizational initiatives to help empower nurses and other healthcare professionals in their workplaces. This clearinghouse provided a singular platform that professionals could use to identify innovative services, research, and networks for their organizations and to access thought leaders engaged in shared governance.

Shortly thereafter, the main website was launched *(www.sharedgovernance.org)*. The Forum for Shared Governance was established as a small endeavor with a singular purpose. However, it has since grown to encompass a global community of researchers, educators, speakers, and practitioners.

The Mission

The central belief of the Forum is that governance innovations can and do enhance patient, organizational, and professional outcomes by empowering staff, managers, and patients to share control and influence over healthcare organizations. The Forum adheres to the idea that staff and managers need ongoing education and support to effectively participate in innovative governance models in those organizations. The mission of the Forum is to support and nurture shared governance within healthcare organizations by providing the community, information, and tools they need.

The Tools

The Forum has grown well beyond the original, narrow concept to become an international clearinghouse for research and resources. Those resources include a growing and supportive shared governance community, as well as tools for implementing and evaluating the measurable impact of shared governance on the organization. Some tools the Forum provides include the following:

Weekly updates

In support of the mission of nurturing shared governance programs, the Forum provides weekly updates on the latest collaborative and independent research, publishing and speaking, and worldwide events, as well as the status of shared governance in specific healthcare organizations.

Q&A advisory board

The Forum website receives questions from staff and managers from all over the world, ranging from those just curious about shared governance to professionals desperate for answers to difficult questions. To help with inquiries, the Forum established an advisory board composed of a "who's who" in shared governance, ranging from iconic thought leaders (e.g., Tim Porter-O'Grady, DM, EdD, ScD[h], FAAN) to healthcare providers whose daily professional lives are intertwined with shared governance through participation in divisionwide and unit-based hospital councils. A number of healthcare providers, leaders, managers, and staff members from all over the U.S. and the globe volunteer to respond to questions posed through the Forum's website, some of which are combined as enduring responses to recurring queries.

Shared governance hospitals online community

One of the ways the Forum supports healthcare staff and managers looking to launch new or reinvigorate weary shared governance programs is by connecting them to a community of established shared governance programs. The SG Hospitals Online section of the website features a list of healthcare organizations promoting themselves through their own public Web pages as having implemented shared governance programs. Visitors can link to the organizations' sites for a more detailed description of their programs and can contact program representatives through email.

The sole criteria for inclusion in this list include the following:
- A public Web page that mentions the shared governance program
- A contact person (credentials, job title, and email address)

Cold calls from those interested in shared governance to those invested have created an informal, organic virtual community of shared governance that has grown to more than a hundred engaged shared governance contacts.

> **A cyber community of participants and researchers in shared governance**
>
> In 2007, the Forum received an email from a hospital representative requesting to be listed on the shared-governance.org website (the SG Hospitals Online page). The sender's email address connected to a Middle Eastern hospital with a stunning online shared governance presence. The Forum requested a contact person for the listing, but weeks and months passed with no response.
>
> Six months later, a second email came through: "Here is our contact person. We're so sorry we have been so tardy in getting back to you. We've been having a war." The email was from the American University of Beirut Medical Center, which shortly thereafter became the first validated shared governance hospital outside of the United States. Even a very real war had not stopped this organization from establishing a stellar shared governance program!

Online research library on shared governance

The Forum's articles site provides access to the only online source of research citations related to shared governance in healthcare. Hundreds of annotated articles are listed for a quick review of the literature, many with direct links to the complete article. This is useful for those writing a grant proposal, capstone project, or hospital-based research plan for an institutional review board (IRB). See Appendix 37 for sample forum articles from 2013.

The Forum's measurement site leads to a complete listing of research that has been conducted with the Index of Professional Nursing Governance (IPNG), which measures governance of nurses in healthcare organizations, and the Index of Professional Governance (IPG), which surveys the perceptions of governance of all professional work groups within an organization (see Appendix A for the IPNG and IPG tools). The collection also includes abstracts of graduate theses, dissertations, and capstone projects that used the tools. Additionally, the Forum's website provides instant access to downloadable PDF versions of the survey instruments at no cost.

The website contains a list of more than 150 organizations in the United States and abroad that have used the IPNG or IPG over the last 20 years to evaluate the implementation of innovative management models and to track changes in governance.

Registered user resources

Those who register on the Forum website gain access to free continuing education as well as periodic discounted material about shared governance, including books. There is no charge, but users must register and create a free member account to access the area of the website that contains these resources.

During the last heyday of shared governance proliferation, which coincided with the last surfeit of nurses, two Miami Valley, Ohio, nurses published the *Journal of Shared Governance*. Although now defunct, past copies can be obtained through this section of the website. The journals are full of still-relevant articles and early research.

Members receive the monthly e-newsletter distributed by the Forum, and have access to posted advice on many topics, such as what to do with petulant participants, how to budget and pay a president of shared governance, and other controversial issues. Registered members also may participate in Bob's Blog, a feature that facilitates collegial exchanges of advice among the expanding community of professionals involved in shared governance research, implementation, and sustainment.

Summary

In summary, healthcare today is in the midst of major global transformations in effectiveness, efficiency, safety, and value. Building registries, evidence-based practices, collaborative relationships, and a strong foundation of research in shared governance is critical for combatting the fragmentation and redundancies in practice and learning environments. Shared governance has become a major factor in the systems redesigns of organizations' operating structures, supporting excellence through interprofessional partnerships, publications, and research. The Forum provides an international clearinghouse of ongoing research, resources, and information to help organizations and their teams at every phase of development and implementation create an efficient and sustainable foundation of practice and excellence in service.

Chapter 12

Conclusions and Recommendations
Where Do We Go From Here?

The future is like heaven;
Everyone exults in it but no one wants to go there now.
        —James Baldwin

Healthcare today is more complex, interrelated, and intersected than ever before as we transition from the industrial age to a socio-technical age (Porter-O'Grady, 2009c):

- Information is exploding as organizations move to digitize all data and transform how healthcare providers communicate and interact with information
- Globalization of the economy is demanding new and different relationships among providers and communities of practice
- Complex and adaptive systems require structurally integrated processes, interactions, and communication pathways
- Hospitals are reducing focus on inpatient activities and increasing focus on quality, safety, and efficiencies
- Constant change demands sustainable, cost-effective services and relationships
- Healthcare services are being reconfigured and merged into integrated service pathways, cross-functional teams, and transformative approaches to leadership
- More effective point-of-service administrative designs, equity-based models with shared decision-making, and knowledge-based ownership of work processes, management support, and consultative roles of interprofessional partners and multidisciplinary team members are being established

- There is growing competition among systems to provide greater cost-effective, safe, high-quality services that increase satisfaction among stakeholders (patients, providers, communities)

Advanced practice nurses, clinical specialists, and healthcare providers with postgraduate degrees in multiple specialties and subspecialties manage their own clinics, work with congregations (e.g., parish nurses), serve on criminology and forensic teams, and support justice departments and attorneys (e.g., legal consultants). They are scientists, researchers, and humanitarians. Healthcare providers serve in the military and practice at all points of service in hospitals, in the home, and in community centers for the homeless and disenfranchised. They are first responders to disasters (hurricanes, floods, and terrorist attacks) and often stay long after others have returned home. Healthcare providers minister to the physical, emotional, psychological, and spiritual needs of humanity of every age, race, culture, and sociopolitical and economic circumstance according to their own scopes of practice. Many providers hold advanced degrees at master's, doctoral, and postdoctoral levels with knowledge and skill in research and evidence-based practice.

Why Shared Governance?

Knowing is not enough; we must apply.
Willing is not enough; we must do.
—Goethe

Shared governance is the present and future of healthcare. It incorporates the qualities and principles needed to operationalize a structure that facilitates full engagement of internal and external stakeholders in complex and adaptive healthcare systems. Leadership and direct-care providers break down old paradigms and frameworks for professional practice. They move processes and systems to an interprofessional, multidisciplinary, integrated, evidence-based infrastructure outward from points of service, resulting in better care outcomes.

Yet implementation of shared governance has made an uneasy journey into professional practice. This work and that of such leaders in shared governance as Tim Porter-O'Grady, Robert Hess (coauthor of this book), and Marla Weston (see Appendix B for bibliographic references) offer some insight into how to continue to reshape and transform healthcare practice through the design and redesign of sustainable systems. Refer to these studies for guidance specific to your organization's history and experience with shared governance:

- When shared governance is newly established (Haag-Heitman and George, 2010; Swihart, 2011; Edmonstone, 2003)
- When shared governance is in early formations, usually within the first three to five years (Hess, 1998a, 1998b, 2009; Porter-O'Grady, 2004, 2009a, 2009b, 2009c)

- When shared governance is well established, usually after the first five years (Porter-O'Grady, 2004, 2009a, 2009b, 2009c; Swihart, 2011; Weston, 2006)
- When shared governance structures and processes are in trouble (Porter-O'Grady and Basinger, 2010; Porter-O'Grady and Hitchings, 2005; Wright, 2005)

Although leaders and interprofessional partners recognize the value of shared governance, nursing has been a primary driving force in implementing this model in healthcare organizations. More recently, research across professions and integration of services have generated a greater interest in shared governance systems from agencies such as the Institute of Medicine (IOM, 2011) and the American Nurses Credentialing Center (Haag-Heitman and George, 2010).

For example, the IOM put forth dramatic observations and recommendations in its report on the future of nursing. In the opening summary, it lays out a strong foundation for implementing shared governance and using an organizational process model within all levels of professional nursing practice as a way to lead change and advance health (2011):

The United States has the opportunity to transform its healthcare system to provide seamless, affordable, quality care that is accessible to all, patient-centered, and evidence-based, and leads to improved health outcomes. Achieving this transformation will require remodeling many aspects of the healthcare system. This is especially true for the nursing profession, the largest segment of the healthcare workforce. This report offers recommendations that collectively serve as a blueprint to (1) ensure that nurses can practice to the full extent of their education and training, (2) improve nursing education, (3) provide opportunities for nurses to assume leadership positions and to serve as full partners in healthcare redesign and improvement efforts, and (4) improve data collection for workforce planning and policy making. (p. 1)

Where Do We Go From Here?

The journey of a thousand miles begins with one step.
—Lao Tzu

A new generation beckons. Lived shared governance is professional practice in action. If the IOM recommendations are "building blocks … to expand innovative models of care … to improve the quality, accessibility, and value of care" (2011, p. 278), then shared governance is an organizational management process model that can transform the current culture of healthcare into one that supports and advances those recommendations in diverse practice settings through professional practice. To create the infrastructure necessary to support and sustain interprofessional shared governance, multiple integrated activities are required:

- Build for growth, progress, and sustainability of shared governance
- Establish and sustain relationships across service lines and within departments

- Develop and sustain transformative leaders, managers, and supervisors
- Select members from across disciplines for the design team (steering group)
- Deploy cross-functional teams and partnerships, especially when setting up practice or unit councils for smaller groups of employees (e.g., clinics)
- Establish integrated communication pathways to enhance communication, relationship-building, accountability, and shared decision-making processes
- Explore the Forum for Shared Governance (*www.sharedgovernance.org*) and the insights, best practices, lessons learned, research, competencies, and evidence-based practices for ideas and resources that might fit into your own structures, processes, and outcomes
- Evaluate processes, momentum, ongoing relevancy, and impact for continual improvement and stakeholder engagement through research and evidence-based practice activities (see Appendix 37 for a collection of shared governance articles and research from 2013)

Healthcare providers facilitate safe, effective, high-quality, and competent service under a plethora of regulatory, business, and organizational conditions and directives. Although the recommendations in the IOM report are directed at policymakers, payers, executives, and other professionals from private and public arenas, they resonate with direct-care nurses and all other healthcare providers. The target audience for the IOM recommendations and conclusions may have the power to change healthcare systems nationally and globally. However, the real transformation begins with providers and staff engaged in genuine shared governance at points of service and the formal involvement of patients and their families.

In Conclusion

Healthcare providers must drive the future of healthcare. Explore the challenges, the possibilities, and the joys that are to come with great purpose and courage. Learn continuously. Integrate processes that prevent duplication, repetition, and redundancy, and facilitate opportunities to grow and build through interprofessional practice and shared governance. Whatever the future of healthcare will be, it begins now, in the present, with us.

Appendix A

Index of Professional Nursing Governance (IPNG)

Index of Professional Governance (IPG)

PROFESSIONAL NURSING GOVERNANCE

Please provide the following information. The information you provide is IMPORTANT. Please be sure to complete ALL questions. Remember confidentiality will be maintained at all times. Today's Date _____

1. Sex: _____ Male _____ Female
2. Age: _____
3. Please indicate your BASIC nursing educational preparation:
   _____ Nursing Diploma _____ Associate Degree in Nursing
   _____ Baccalaureate Degree in Nursing
4. Please indicate the HIGHEST educational degree that you have attained at this point in time:
   _____ Nursing Diploma _____ Master's Degree, Non-nursing
   _____ Associate Degree in Nursing _____ Doctorate, Nursing
   _____ Baccalaureate Degree in Nursing _____ Doctorate, Non-nursing
   _____ Master's Degree in Nursing, Specialty
5. Employment Status:
   _____ Full-time, 36-40 hours per week
   _____ Part-time, less than 36 hours per week (specify number of hours/week): _____
6. Please specify the number of years that you have been practicing nursing _____
7. Please indicate the title of your present position _____
8. Please indicate the type of nursing unit that you work on:
   _____ Medical   _____ Maternity
   _____ Surgical   _____ Pediatrics
   _____ Critical Care   _____ Psychiatry
   _____ Operating Room _____ Education
   _____ Recovery Room   _____ Quality Management
   _____ Emergency Room _____ Outside Nursing
   _____ Clinic   _____ Other (please specify): _____
9. Please specify the number of years you have worked in this institution _____
10. Please specify the number of years you have been in this present position _____
11. Have you received any specialty certifications from professional organizations? _____ Yes _____ No
    If YES, please specify the type of certification and year received _____

In your organization, please circle the group that CONTROLS the following areas:

1 = Nursing management/administration only
2 = Primarily nursing management/administration with some staff nurse input
3 = Equally shared by staff nurses and nursing management/administration
4 = Primarily staff nurses with some nursing management/administration input
5 = Staff nurses only

PART I

1. Determining what nurses can do at the bedside. | 1 | 2 | 3 | 4 | 5
2. Developing and evaluating policies, procedures and protocols related to patient care. | 1 | 2 | 3 | 4 | 5
3. Establishing levels of qualifications for nursing positions. | 1 | 2 | 3 | 4 | 5
4. Evaluating nursing personnel (performance appraisals and peer review). | 1 | 2 | 3 | 4 | 5
5. Determining activities of ancillary nursing personnel (assistants, technicians, secretaries). | 1 | 2 | 3 | 4 | 5
6. Conducting disciplinary action of nursing personnel. | 1 | 2 | 3 | 4 | 5
7. Assessing and providing for the professional/educational development of the nursing staff. | 1 | 2 | 3 | 4 | 5
8. Making hiring decisions about RNs and other nursing personnel. | 1 | 2 | 3 | 4 | 5
9. Promoting RNs and other nursing personnel. | 1 | 2 | 3 | 4 | 5
10. Appointing nursing personnel to management and leadership positions. | 1 | 2 | 3 | 4 | 5
11. Selecting products used in nursing care. | 1 | 2 | 3 | 4 | 5
12. Incorporating evidence-based practice into nursing care. | 1 | 2 | 3 | 4 | 5
13. Determining models of nursing care delivery (e.g. primary, team). | 1 | 2 | 3 | 4 | 5

© 1998, 2013 Robert G. Hess, Jr., RN, PhD. To obtain permission for use, call (856) 424-4270 or e-mail info@sharedgovernance.org.

PROFESSIONAL NURSING GOVERNANCE

In your organization, please circle the group that influences the following activities:

1 = Nursing management/administration only
2 = Primarily nursing management/administration with some staff nurse input
3 = Equally shared by staff nurses and nursing management/administration
4 = Primarily staff nurses with some nursing management/administration input
5 = Staff nurses only

PART II

14. Determining how many and what level of nursing staff is needed for routine patient care. 1 2 3 4 5
15. Adjusting staffing levels to meet fluctuations in patient census and acuity. 1 2 3 4 5
16. Making daily patient care assignments for nursing personnel. 1 2 3 4 5
17. Monitoring and procuring supplies for nursing care and support functions. 1 2 3 4 5
18. Regulating the flow of patient admissions, transfers, and discharges. 1 2 3 4 5
19. Formulating annual unit budgets for personnel, supplies, equipment and education. 1 2 3 4 5
20. Recommending nursing salaries, raises and benefits. 1 2 3 4 5
21. Consulting and enlisting the support of nursing services outside of the unit (e.g. clinical experts such as psychiatric or wound care specialists, diabetic educators). 1 2 3 4 5
22. Consulting and enlisting the support of services outside of nursing (e.g. dietary, social service, pharmacy, human resources, finance). 1 2 3 4 5
23. Making recommendations concerning other departments' resources. 1 2 3 4 5
24. Determining cost-effective measures such as patient placement and referrals or supply management (e.g. placement of ventilator-dependent patients, early discharge of patients to home health care). 1 2 3 4 5
25. Recommending new services or specialties (e.g. gerontology, mental health, birthing centers). 1 2 3 4 5
26. Creating new clinical positions. 1 2 3 4 5
27. Creating new administrative or support positions. 1 2 3 4 5

According to the following indicators in your organization, please circle which group has OFFICIAL AUTHORITY (i.e. authority granted and recognized by the organization) over the following areas that control practice and influence the resources that support it:

1 = Nursing management/administration only
2 = Primarily nursing management/administration with some staff nurse input
3 = Equally shared by staff nurses and nursing management/administration
4 = Primarily staff nurses with some nursing management/administration input
5 = Staff nurses only

PART III

28. Written policies and procedures that state what nurses can do related to direct patient care. 1 2 3 4 5
29. Written patient care standard/protocols and quality assurance/improvement processes. 1 2 3 4 5
30. Mandatory RN credentialing levels (licensure, education, certifications) for hiring, continued employment, promotions and raises. 1 2 3 4 5
31. Written process for evaluating nursing personnel (performance appraisal, peer review). 1 2 3 4 5
32. Organizational charts that show job titles and who reports to whom. 1 2 3 4 5
33. Written guidelines for disciplining nursing personnel. 1 2 3 4 5
34. Annual requirements for continuing education and inservices. 1 2 3 4 5
35. Procedures for hiring and transferring nursing personnel. 1 2 3 4 5
36. Policies regulating promotion of nursing personnel to management and leadership positions. 1 2 3 4 5
37. Procedures for generating schedules for RNs and other nursing staff. 1 2 3 4 5
38. Acuity and/or patient classification systems for determining how many and what level of nursing staff is needed for routine patient care. 1 2 3 4 5

PROFESSIONAL NURSING GOVERNANCE

39. Mechanisms for determining staffing levels when there are fluctuations in patient census and acuity. 1 2 3 4 5

40. Procedures for determining daily patient care assignments. 1 2 3 4 5

41. Daily methods for monitoring and obtaining supplies for nursing care and support functions. 1 2 3 4 5

42. Procedures for controlling the flow of patient admissions, transfers and discharges. 1 2 3 4 5

43. Process for recommending and formulating annual unit budgets for personnel, supplies, major equipment and education. 1 2 3 4 5

44. Procedures for adjusting nursing salaries, raises and benefits. 1 2 3 4 5

45. Formal mechanisms for consulting and enlisting the support of nursing services outside of the unit. (e.g. clinical experts such as psychiatric or wound care specialists, diabetic educators). 1 2 3 4 5

46. Formal mechanisms for consulting and enlisting the support of services outside of nursing. (e.g. dietary, social service, pharmacy, human resources, finance). 1 2 3 4 5

47. Procedure for restricting or limiting patient care (e.g. closing hospital beds, going on ER bypass). 1 2 3 4 5

48. Location, design and access to office space, staff lounges and charting areas. 1 2 3 4 5

49. Access to office equipment (e.g. smart phones, computers, copy machines) and the Internet. 1 2 3 4 5

In your hospital, please circle the group that PARTICIPATES in the following activities:

1 = Nursing management/administration only
2 = Primarily nursing management/administration with some staff nurse input
3 = Equally shared by staff nurses and nursing management/administration
4 = Primarily staff nurses with some nursing management/administration input
5 = Staff nurses only

PART IV

50. Participation in unit committees for clinical practice. 1 2 3 4 5

51. Participation in unit committees for administrative matters, such as staffing, scheduling and budgeting. 1 2 3 4 5

52. Participation in nursing departmental committees for clinical practice. 1 2 3 4 5

53. Participation in nursing departmental committees for administrative matters such as staffing, scheduling, and budgeting. 1 2 3 4 5

54. Participation in interprofessional committees (physicians, other healthcare professions and departments) for collaborative practice. 1 2 3 4 5

55. Participation in hospital administration committees for matters such as employee benefits and strategic planning. 1 2 3 4 5

56. Forming new unit committees. 1 2 3 4 5

57. Forming new nursing departmental committees. 1 2 3 4 5

58. Forming new interprofessional committees. 1 2 3 4 5

59. Forming new administration committees for the organization. 1 2 3 4 5

PROFESSIONAL NURSING GOVERNANCE

In your organization, please circle the group that has Access to information about the following activities:

1 = Nursing management/administration only
2 = Primarily nursing management/administration with some staff nurse input
3 = Equally shared by staff nurses and nursing management/administration
4 = Primarily staff nurses with some nursing management/administration input
5 = Staff nurses only

PART V

60. The quality of nursing practice in the organization. 1 2 3 4 5
61. Compliance of nursing practice with requirements of surveying agencies (The Joint Commission, state and federal government, professional groups). 1 2 3 4 5
62. Unit's projected budget and actual expenses. 1 2 3 4 5
63. Organization's financial status. 1 2 3 4 5
64. Unit and nursing departmental goals and objectives for this year. 1 2 3 4 5
65. Organization's strategic plans for the next few years. 1 2 3 4 5
66. Results of patient satisfaction surveys. 1 2 3 4 5
67. Physician/nurse satisfaction with their collaborative practice. 1 2 3 4 5
68. Current status of nurse turnover and vacancies in the organization. 1 2 3 4 5
69. Nurses' satisfaction with their general practice. 1 2 3 4 5
70. Nurses' satisfaction with their salaries and benefits. 1 2 3 4 5
71. Management's opinion of the quality of bedside nursing practice. 1 2 3 4 5
72. Physicians' opinion of the quality of bedside nursing practice. 1 2 3 4 5
73. Nursing peers' opinion of the quality of bedside nursing practice. 1 2 3 4 5
74. Access to resources supporting professional practice and development (e.g. online resources, CE activities, journals and books, library). 1 2 3 4 5

In your hospital, please circle the group that has the ABILITY to:

1 = Nursing management/administration only
2 = Primarily nursing management/administration with some staff nurse input
3 = Equally shared by staff nurses and nursing management/administration
4 = Primarily staff nurses with some nursing management/administration input
5 = Staff nurses only

PART VI

75. Negotiate solutions to conflicts among professional nurses. 1 2 3 4 5
76. Negotiate solutions to conflicts between professional nurses and physicians. 1 2 3 4 5
77. Negotiate solutions to conflicts between professional nurses and other healthcare services (respiratory, dietary, etc). 1 2 3 4 5
78. Negotiate solutions to conflicts between professional nurses and nursing management. 1 2 3 4 5
79. Negotiate solutions to conflicts between professional nurses and the organization's administration. 1 2 3 4 5
80. Create a formal grievance procedure or a process for resolving internal disputes. 1 2 3 4 5
81. Write the goals and objectives of a nursing unit. 1 2 3 4 5
82. Write the philosophy, goals and objectives of the nursing department. 1 2 3 4 5
83. Formulate the mission, philosophy, goals and objectives of the organization. 1 2 3 4 5
84. Write unit policies and procedures. 1 2 3 4 5
85. Determine nursing departmental policies and procedures. 1 2 3 4 5
86. Determine organization-wide policies and procedures. 1 2 3 4 5

PROFESSIONAL GOVERNANCE

Please provide the following information. The information you provide is IMPORTANT. Please be sure to complete ALL questions. Remember confidentiality will be maintained at all times. Today's Date _____

1. Sex: ____ Male ____ Female
2. Age: ____
3. Please indicate your profession:
   ____ Accountant   ____ Physician
   ____ Dietician   ____ Registered Nurse
   ____ Pharmacist   ____ Respiratory Therapist
   ____ Physical Therapist ____ Social Worker
   ____ Other
4. Please indicate your HIGHEST educational degree:
   ____ Diploma   ____ Master's Degree
   ____ Associate Degree   ____ Doctorate
   ____ Baccalaureate Degree
5. Employment Status:
   ____ Full-time, 36–40 hours per week
   ____ Part-time, less than 36 hours per week (specify number of hours/week): ____
6. Please specify the number of years that you have been practicing ____
7. Please indicate the title of your present position ____
8. Please indicate your clinical specialty:
   ____ Case Management   ____ Maternity   ____ Psychiatry
   ____ Clinic   ____ Medical/Surgical ____ Quality Management
   ____ Critical Care   ____ Operating Room   ____ Recovery Room
   ____ Education   ____ Pediatrics   ____ Rehabilitation
   ____ Emergency Room   ____ Other (specify): ____
9. Please specify the number of years you have worked in this organization ____
10. Please specify the number of years you have been in your present position ____
11. Please rate your overall satisfaction with your professional practice within the organization (1 = lowest, 5 = highest):   1   2   3   4   5

In your organization, please circle the group that CONTROLS the following areas:

1 = Management/administration only
2 = Primarily management/administration with some staff input
3 = Equally shared by staff and management/administration
4 = Primarily staff with some management/administration input
5 = Staff only

PART I

1. Determining what your professional colleagues can do in their daily practice.   1 2 3 4 5
2. Developing and evaluating policies, procedures and protocols related to patient care.   1 2 3 4 5
3. Establishing levels of qualifications for positions within your own discipline.   1 2 3 4 5
4. Evaluating professional personnel within your own discipline (performance appraisals and peer review).   1 2 3 4 5
5. Determining activities of ancillary personnel (aides, assistants, technicians, secretaries).   1 2 3 4 5
6. Conducting disciplinary actions of colleagues within your discipline.   1 2 3 4 5
7. Assessing and providing for the professional/educational development of professionals within your own discipline.   1 2 3 4 5
8. Making hiring decisions about professionals within your discipline and their support staff.   1 2 3 4 5
9. Promoting colleagues and their support staff.   1 2 3 4 5
10. Appointing personnel to management and leadership positions.   1 2 3 4 5
11. Selecting products used in your professional practice.   1 2 3 4 5
12. Incorporating evidence-based practice into your professional practice.   1 2 3 4 5
13. Determining methods or systems for accomplishing the work of your discipline.   1 2 3 4 5

© 1998, 2013 Robert G. Hess, Jr., RN, PhD. To obtain permission for use, call (856) 424-4270 or e-mail info@sharedgovernance.org.

PROFESSIONAL GOVERNANCE

In your organization, please circle the group that INFLUENCES the following activities:

1 = Management/administration only
2 = Primarily management/administration with some staff input
3 = Equally shared by staff and management/administration
4 = Primarily staff with some management/administration input
5 = Staff only

PART II

14. Determining how many staff and what level of expertise is needed for routine work. 1 2 3 4 5
15. Adjusting staffing levels to meet fluctuations in work demands. 1 2 3 4 5
16. Making work assignments for professional and support staff. 1 2 3 4 5
17. Monitoring and procuring supplies necessary for professional practice and support functions. 1 2 3 4 5
18. Regulating the flow of services or patients/clients within the organization. 1 2 3 4 5
19. Formulating annual unit budgets for personnel, supplies, equipment, and education for your own unit or work group. 1 2 3 4 5
20. Recommending salaries, raises and benefits. 1 2 3 4 5
21. Consulting and enlisting services outside of your own unit or work group. 1 2 3 4 5
22. Consulting and enlisting the support of services outside of your own discipline (e.g. dietary, social service, pharmacy, human resources, finance). 1 2 3 4 5
23. Making recommendations concerning other departments' resources. 1 2 3 4 5
24. Determining cost-effective measures for professional practice. 1 2 3 4 5
25. Recommending new services or ventures. 1 2 3 4 5
26. Creating new clinical positions. 1 2 3 4 5
27. Creating new administrative or support positions. 1 2 3 4 5

According to the following indicators in your organization, please circle which group has OFFICIAL AUTHORITY (i.e. authority granted and recognized by the organization) over the following areas that control practice and influence the resources that support it:

1 = Management/administration only
2 = Primarily management/administration with some staff input
3 = Equally shared by staff and management/administration
4 = Primarily staff with some management/administration input
5 = Staff only

PART III

28. Written policies and procedures that state what activities professional colleagues can related to their daily practice. 1 2 3 4 5
29. Written service standards/protocols and quality improvement processes. 1 2 3 4 5
30. Mandatory credentialing levels of professionals (licensure, education, certifications) for hiring, continued employment, promotions and raises. 1 2 3 4 5
31. Written process for evaluating professional personnel within your own discipline (performance appraisal, peer review). 1 2 3 4 5
32. Organizational charts that show job titles and who reports to whom. 1 2 3 4 5
33. Written guidelines for disciplining personnel. 1 2 3 4 5
34. Annual requirements for continuing education and inservices. 1 2 3 4 5
35. Procedures for hiring and transferring your discipline's personnel. 1 2 3 4 5
36. Policies regulating promotion of professional personnel to management and leadership positions. 1 2 3 4 5
37. Procedures for generating schedules for professionals within your own discipline and their support staff. 1 2 3 4 5

© 2014 HCPro

PROFESSIONAL GOVERNANCE

In your organization, please circle the group that PARTICIPATES in the following activities:

1 = Management/administration only
2 = Primarily management/administration with some staff input
3 = Equally shared by staff and management/administration
4 = Primarily staff with some management/administration input
5 = Staff only

38. Systems for determining how many staff and what level of expertise is needed for the day-to-day work of your unit or work group.   1   2   3   4   5

39. Mechanisms for determining staffing levels when there are fluctuations in work demands.   1   2   3   4   5

40. Procedures for determining work assignments.   1   2   3   4   5

41. Daily methods for monitoring and obtaining supplies that support the practice of your professional group within the organization.   1   2   3   4   5

42. Procedures for controlling the flow of services and patients/clients within the organization.   1   2   3   4   5

42. Process for recommending and formulating annual budgets for personnel, supplies, equipment, and education for your own work group.   1   2   3   4   5

44. Procedures for adjusting professional personnel's salaries, raises, and benefits.   1   2   3   4   5

45. Formal mechanisms for consulting and enlisting the support of other professionals within your discipline who work outside of your work group.   1   2   3   4   5

46. Formal mechanisms for consulting and enlisting support of organizational services outside of your work group (e.g. dietary, social service, pharmacy, human resources, finance).   1   2   3   4   5

47. Procedure for restricting or limiting the amount of work you do (closing units, redistributing patient work loads).   1   2   3   4   5

48. Location, design and access to office space, staff lounges and charting areas.   1   2   3   4   5

49. Access to office equipment (e.g. smart phones, computers, copy machines) and the Internet.   1   2   3   4   5

PART IV

50. Participation in unit or work-group committees that deal with professional practice.   1   2   3   4   5

51. Participation in unit or work-group committees that deal with administrative matters such as staffing, scheduling and budgeting.   1   2   3   4   5

52. Participation in departmental committees that deal with professional practice.   1   2   3   4   5

52. Participation in departmental committees that deal with administrative matters such as staffing, scheduling, and budgeting.   1   2   3   4   5

54. Participation in interprofessional committees (physicians, other healthcare professions) for collaborative practice.   1   2   3   4   5

55. Participation in organizational administrative committees for matters such as employee benefits and strategic planning.   1   2   3   4   5

56. Formating new unit or work-group committees.   1   2   3   4   5

57. Forming new departmental committees within your own discipline.   1   2   3   4   5

58. Forming new interprofessional committees.   1   2   3   4   5

59. Forming new administration committees for the organization.   1   2   3   4   5

© 2014 HCPro

PROFESSIONAL GOVERNANCE

In your organization, please circle the group that has ACCESS TO INFORMATION about the following activities:

1 = Management/administration only
2 = Primarily management/administration with some staff input
3 = Equally shared by staff and management/administration
4 = Primarily staff with some management/administration input
5 = Staff only

PART V

#	Item	1	2	3	4	5
60.	Quality of professional practice in the organization.	1	2	3	4	5
61.	Compliance of your organization with requirements of surveying agencies (e.g. The Joint Commission, state and federal government, professional groups).	1	2	3	4	5
62.	Your work group's projected budget and actual expenses.	1	2	3	4	5
63.	Your organization's financial status.	1	2	3	4	5
64.	Your work group and departmental goals and objectives for this year.	1	2	3	4	5
65.	Your organization's strategic plans for the next few years.	1	2	3	4	5
66.	Results of clients' satisfaction surveys.	1	2	3	4	5
67.	Professionals' satisfaction with their interprofessional collaboration.	1	2	3	4	5
68.	Turnover and vacancy rate of professionals within your discipline in the organization.	1	2	3	4	5
69.	Colleagues' (within your discipline) satisfaction with their general practice.	1	2	3	4	5
70.	Colleagues' (within your discipline) satisfaction with their salaries and benefits.	1	2	3	4	5
71.	Management's opinion of the quality of professional practice provided by your discipline.	1	2	3	4	5
72.	Other professional disciplines' opinion of the quality of professional practice provided by your discipline.	1	2	3	4	5
73.	Your peers' opinion of the quality of their professional practice.	1	2	3	4	5
74.	Access to resources supporting professional practice and development (e.g. online resources, CE activities, journals and books library).	1	2	3	4	5

In your organization, please circle the group that has the ABILITY to:

1 = Management/administration only
2 = Primarily management/administration with some staff input
3 = Equally shared by staff and management/administration
4 = Primarily staff with some management/administration input
5 = Staff only

PART VI

#	Item	1	2	3	4	5
75.	Negotiate solutions to conflicts among your professional colleagues.	1	2	3	4	5
76.	Negotiate solutions to conflicts between your professional colleagues and other professional groups.	1	2	3	4	5
77.	Negotiate solutions to conflicts between your professional colleagues and other organizational departments.	1	2	3	4	5
78.	Negotiate solutions to conflicts between your professional colleagues and their immediate managers.	1	2	3	4	5
79.	Negotiate solutions to conflicts between your professional colleagues and the organization's administration.	1	2	3	4	5
80.	Create a formal grievance procedure or process for resolving internal disputes.	1	2	3	4	5
81.	Write the goals and objectives for your immediate work group.	1	2	3	4	5
82.	Write the philosophy, goals, and objectives of your department.	1	2	3	4	5
83.	Formulate the mission, philosophy, goals, and objectives of the organization.	1	2	3	4	5
84.	Write policies and procedures for your work group.	1	2	3	4	5
85.	Determine departmental policies and procedures.	1	2	3	4	5
86.	Determine organization-wide policies and procedures.	1	2	3	4	5

Appendix B
Expanded Bibliography

Allen, D., Calkin, J., & Peterson, M. (1988). Making shared governance work: A conceptual model. *Journal of Nursing Administration* 18(1): 37–43.

Alvarado, K., Boblin-Cummings, S., & Goddard, P. (2000). Experiencing nursing governance: Developing a post merger nursing committee structure. *Canadian Journal of Nursing Leadership* 13(4): 30–35.

American Association of Colleges of Nursing. (2002). *AACN White Paper: Hallmarks of the Professional Nursing Practice Environment.* Washington, DC: Author.

American Hospital Association. (2002). *How Hospital Leaders can Build a Thriving Workforce.* Washington, DC: AHA Commission on Workforce for Hospitals and Health Systems.

American Hospital Association. (2010). Fast facts on US hospitals. Retrieved March 20, 2011, from *www.aha.org/aha/resource-center/Statistics-and-Studies/fast-facts.html.*

American National Standards Institute/International Organization for Standardization/ASQ(E)Q9001-2008 (2008). American National Standard, Quality Management System Requirements. Milwaukee: American Society for Quality.

American Nurses Association. (2001a). *ANA's Bill of Rights for Registered Nurses.* Washington, DC: Author.

American Nurses Association. (2001b). *Code of Ethics for Nurses, with Interpretive Statements.* Washington, DC: Author.

American Nurses Association. (2003). ANA reorganizes structure to better meet nurses' needs. *The American Nurse* 35(4): 12–13.

American Nurses Association. (2004). *Scope and Standards for Nurse Administrators* (2nd ed.). Washington, DC: Author.

American Nurses Association. (2005). Principles for nurse staffing. In *Utilization Guide for the ANA Principles for Nurse Staffing* (pp. 20–28). Silver Spring, MD: Author.

American Nurses Association. (2010). *Nursing Professional Development: Scope and Standards of Practice.* Washington, DC: Author.

American Nurses Credentialing Center. (2004). *Magnet Recognition Program®: Application Manual 2005.* Silver Spring, MD: Author.

American Nurses Credentialing Center. (2008). *Magnet Recognition Program®: Application Manual.* Silver Spring, MD: Author.

American Nurses Credentialing Center. (2008). *The Magnet Model Components and Sources of Evidence: Magnet Recognition Program®.* Silver Spring, MD: Author.

American Nurses Credentialing Center. (2011). ISO journey at ANCC. Retrieved April 10, 2014, from *www.nursecredentialing.org/FunctionalCategory/AboutANCC/ISOJourney.aspx.*

American Organization of Nurse Executives. (2000). *Perspectives on the nursing shortage: A blueprint for action.* Chicago, IL: AONE.

Anderson, B. (1992). Voyage to shared governance. *Nursing Management* 23(11): 65–67.

Anderson, E. (2000). *Empowerment, Job Satisfaction, and Professional Governance of Nurses in Hospitals With and Without Shared Governance.* Doctoral dissertation. New Orleans: School of Nursing, Louisiana State University Medical Center.

Anthony, M. K. (2004). Shared governance models: The theory, practice, and evidence. *Online Journal of Issues in Nursing* 9(1/4).

Arbinger Institute. (2002). *Leadership and Self-Deception: Getting Out of the Box.* San Francisco: Berrett-Koehler Publishers, Inc.

Arter, D. R., & Russell, J. P. (2009). *ISO Lesson Guide 2008: Pocket Guide to ISO 9001-2008* (3rd ed.). Milwaukee: ASQ Quality Press.

Barden, A. M. (2009). *Shared Governance and Empowerment in Nurses Working in a Hospital Setting.* Doctoral dissertation. Cleveland: Case Western Reserve University.

Barker, A. M., Sullivan, D. T., & Emery, M. J. (2006). *Leadership Competencies for Clinical Managers: The Renaissance of Transformational Leadership.* Sudbury, MA: Jones and Bartlett Publishers.

Benner, P. (1984). *From Novice to Expert: Excellence and Power in Clinical Nursing Practice.* Menlo Park, CA: Addison-Wesley Publishing Company.

Beyea, S. C., & Slattery, M. J. (2006). *Evidence-Based Practice in Nursing: A Guide to Successful Implementation.* Marblehead, MA: HCPro, Inc.

Black, J. S., & Gregersen, H. B. (2008). *It Starts with One: Changing Individuals Changes Organizations.* Upper Saddle River, NJ: Prentice Hall.

Blanchard, K., & Hodges, P. (2003). *The Servant-Leader: Transforming Your Heart, Head, Hands & Habits.* Nashville: J. Countryman®, a division of Thomas Nelson, Inc.

Brennan, P. F., & Anthony, M. K. (2000). Measuring nursing practice models using multi-attribute utility theory. *Research in Nursing and Health* 23: 372–382.

Brooks, S. B., Olsen, P., Rieger-Kligys, S., & Mooney, L. (1995). Peer review: An approach to performance evaluation in a professional practice model. *Critical Care Nursing Quarterly* 18(3): 36–47.

Buckingham, M., & Coffman, C. (1999). *First, Break All the Rules: What the World's Greatest Managers Do Differently.* New York: Simon and Schuster.

Burns, J. (1978). *Leadership.* New York: Harper & Row.

Burns, N., & Grove, S. K. (2005). *The Practice of Nursing Research: Conduct, Critique, and Utilization* (5th ed.). St Louis: Elsevier.

Cashman, K. (1998). *Leadership From the Inside Out: Becoming a Leader for Life.* Provo, UT: Executive Excellence Publishing.

Centers for Medicare & Medicaid Services. (2006). *Revised Long-Term-Care Facility Resident Assessment Instrument User's Manual* (Version 2.0, rev). Washington, DC: U.S. Department of Health and Human Services & Author.

Clavelle, J.T., Porter-O'Grady, T., Drenkard, K. (2013). Structural Empowerment and the Nursing Practice Environment in Magnet Organizations. *Journal of Nursing Administration* 43(11): 566–573.

Corley, M. C., Minick, P., Elswick, R. K., & Jacobs, M. (2005). Nurse moral distress and ethical work environment. *Nursing Ethics* 12(4): 382–390.

Cottrell, D., & Adams, A. (2006). *The Next Level: Leading Beyond the Status Quo.* Dallas: CornerStone Leadership Institute.

Covey, S. R. (1991). *Principle-Centered Leadership.* New York: Summit Books.

Daugherty, J., & Hart, P. (1993). Shared governance. *Nursing Management* 24(4): 100–101.

DeBaca, V., Jones, K., & Tornabeni, J. (1993). A cost-benefit analysis of shared governance. *Journal of Nursing Administration* 23(7/8): 50–57.

Donabedian, A. (1980). *The Definition of Quality and Approaches to its Assessment.* Ann Arbor, MI: Health Administration Press.

Donabedian, A. (2003). *An Introduction to Quality Assurance in Health Care.* New York: Oxford University Press.

Dunham-Taylor, J. (2000). Nurse executive transformational leadership found in participative organizations. *Journal of Nursing Administration* 30(5): 241–250.

Eder, S. (2014). *In Focus: A multidisciplinary approach to instrument availability.* Retrieved from *http://dx.doi.org/10.1016/S0001-2092(14)00289-0* at AORN, Inc.

Edmonstone, J. (2003). *Shared Governance: Making It Work.* Chichester, West Sussex, United Kingdom: Kingsham Press.

Evan, K., Aubry, K., Hawkins, M., Curley, T. A., & Porter-O'Grady, T. (1995). Whole systems shared governance: A model for the integrated health system. *Journal of Nursing Administration* 25(5): 18–27.

Farquharson, J. M. (2004). Liability of the nurse manager. In T. D. Aiken (Ed.), *Legal, Ethical, and Political Issues in Nursing* (2nd ed.) (pp. 311–336). Philadelphia: F.A. Davis Company.

Finkler, S. A., Kovner, C. T., Knickman, J. R., & Hendrickson, G. (1994). Innovation in nursing: A benefit/cost analysis. *Nursing Economic$* 12(1): 18–27.

Gardner, D., & Cummings, C. (1994). Total quality management and shared governance: Synergistic processes. *Nursing Administration Quarterly* 18(4): 56–64.

George, V. M., Burke, L. J., & Rodgers, B. L. (1997). Research-based planning for change: Assessing nurses' attitudes toward governance and professional practice autonomy after hospital acquisition. *Journal of Nursing Administration* 27(5): 53–61.

George, V., & Maricarmen, L. (2014). Professional governance: To act—not just inform. *Nurse Leader* 12(2), 48–54.

Green, A., & Jordan, C. (2004). Common denominators: shared governance and work place advocacy—strategies for nurses to gain control over their practice. *Online Journal of Issues in Nursing* 9(1). Retrieved May 14, 2011 from *www.medscape.com/viewarticle/490770*.

Greenhalgh, T. (2004). Diffusion of innovations in service organizations: Systematic review and recommendations. *The Milbank Quarterly* 82: 581–629.

Greenleaf, R. K. (1991, 2008). *The Servant as Leader*. Westfield, IN: The Greenleaf Center for Servant Leadership.

Griffith, J. R., & White, K. R. (2002). *The Well-Managed Healthcare Organization* (5th ed.). Chicago: Health Administration Press.

Haag-Heitman, B., & George, V. (2010). *Guide for Establishing Shared Governance: A Starter's Toolkit*. Silver Spring, MD: American Nurses Credentialing Center. (Entire IPNG and IPG included.)

Havens, D. S., & Aiken, L. H. (1999). Shaping systems to promote desired outcomes: The Magnet hospital model. *Journal of Nursing Administration* 29: 14–20.

Havens, D. S., & Vasey J. (2003). Measuring staff nurse decisional involvement. *Journal of Nursing Administration* 33(6): 331–336.

Hess, R. G. (1994a). Reputational shared governance. *Journal of Nursing Administration* 24(4): 9, 15.

Hess, R. G. (1994b). Shared governance: Innovation or imitation? *Nursing Economic$* 12(1): 28–34.

Hess, R. G. (1995). Shared governance: Nursing's 21st century tower of Babel. *Journal of Nursing Administration* 25(5): 14–17.

Hess, R. G. (1996a). Connecting the dots. Guest editorial. *Journal of Shared Governance* 2(3): 5–8.

Hess, R. G. (1996b). Measuring shared governance outcomes. *Nursing Economic$* 14(4): 254.

Hess, R. G. (1998a). A breed apart—real shared governance. *Journal of Shared Governance* 4(3): 5–6.

Hess, R. G. (1998b). Measuring nursing governance. *Nursing Research* 47(1): 35–42.

Hess, R. G. (2013). From bedside to boardroom—nursing shared governance. *Online Journal of Issues in Nursing*, 9(1). Retrieved May 1, 2013, from *http://ananursece.healthstream.com/*. (NOTE: This is a continuing education program that is updated regularly.)

Hess, R. G. (ND). Petulant participants. Advice from the Forum for Shared Governance. Accessed May 14, 2011 at *www.sharedgovernance.org/PetulantParticipants.htm*.

Hinshaw, A. S. (2002). Building magnetism into health organizations. In M. L. McClure & A. S. Hinshaw (Eds.), *Magnet Hospitals Revisited: Attraction and Retention of Professional Nurses* (pp. 83–102). Washington, DC: American Nurses Association.

Howell, J., Frederick, J., Ollinger, B., Hess, R., & Clipp, E. C. (2001). Can nurses govern in a government agency? *Journal of Nursing Administration* 31: 187–195.

Institute of Health. (2011). Description of patient-centered care. Accessed March 27, 2011 at *www.ihi.org/IHI/Topics/PatientCenteredCare/PatientCenteredCareGeneral/*.

Institute of Medicine. (2001). *Crossing the Quality Chasm*. Washington, DC: National Academies Press.

Institute of Medicine. (2003). *Health Professions Education. A Bridge to Quality*. Washington, DC: National Academies Press.

Institute of Medicine. (2011). *The Future of Nursing: Leading Change, Advancing Health*. Washington, DC: National Academies Press.

Ireson, C., & McGillis, G. (1998). A multidisciplinary shared governance model. *Nursing Management* 29(2): 37–39.

ISO Consultants for Healthcare. (November, 2010). ISO9001:2008 lead auditor for international quality management systems with applications for healthcare. Dayton, OH: ISO Consultants for Healthcare (ICH). For questions or more information, please contact: Ted Schmidt, Chris Kolb, or William J. Metzcar, Executive Oversight, Det Norske Veritas Surveyor, at *wmetzcar@isoforhealthcare.com*.

Jones, G. (2004). *Organizational Theory, Design, and Change* (4th ed.). Upper Saddle River, NJ: Pearson, Prentice Hall.

Jones, L. S., & Ortiz, M. (1989). Increasing nursing autonomy and recognition through shared governance. *Nursing Administration Quarterly* 13(4): 11–16.

Kang, S. (1995). *A Comparison of Shared Governance and Nursing Unit Culture in Three Hospitals*. Master's thesis. Seoul, Korea: Yonsei University.

Keith, K. M. (2008). *The Case for Servant-Leadership*. Westfield, IN: The Greenleaf Center for Servant Leadership.

Kohn, L. T., Corrigan, J. M., & Donaldson, M. S. (Eds.) (1999). *To Err is Human: Building a Safer Health System*. Washington, DC: National Academy Press.

Koloroutis, M. (Ed.) (2004). *Relationship-Based Care: A Model for Transforming Practice.* Minneapolis: Creative Health Care Management.

Kovner, C. T., Hendrickson, G., Knickman, J. R., & Finkler, S. A. (1993). Changing the delivery of nursing care: Implementation issues and qualitative findings. *Journal of Nursing Administration* 23(11): 24–34.

Larkin, M. E., Cierpial, C. L., Stack, J. M., Morrison, V. J., & Griffith, C. A. (March 2008). Empowerment theory in action: The wisdom of collaborative governance. *The Online Journal of Issues in Nursing* 13, 2. Retrieved March 20, 2011, from *www.nursingworld.org/MainMenuCategories/ANAMarketplace/ANAPeriodicals/OJIN/ TableofContents/vol132008/No2May08/ArticlePreviousTopic/EmpowermentTheory.aspx*

Laschinger, H. A. (1996). A theoretical approach to studying work empowerment in nursing: A review of studies testing Kanter's theory of structural power in organizations. *Nursing Administration Quarterly* 20(2), 25–41.

Laschinger, H. K. S., Almost, J., & Tuer-Hodes, D. (2003). Workplace empowerment and magnet hospital characteristics. *Journal of Nursing Administration* 33(7/8): 410–422.

Laschinger, H. K. S., & Havens, D. S. (1996). Staff nurse empowerment and perceived control over nursing practice. *Journal of Nursing Administration* 26(9): 27–35.

Laschinger, H. K. S., Sabiston, J. A., & Kutszcher, L. (1997). Empowerment and staff nurse decision involvement in nursing work environment: Testing Kanter's theory of structural power in organizations. *Research in Nursing and Health* 20: 341–352.

Laschinger, H. K. S., Wong, C., McMahon, L., & Kaufman, C. (1999). Leader behavior impact on staff nurse empowerment, job tension, and work effectiveness. *Journal of Nursing Administration* 29(5): 28–39.

Lee, C., Yang, K., Wu, S., & Lee, L. (2001). The effectiveness of implementing a unit-based shared governance model [Chinese]. *Journal of Nursing Research* (China) 9(2): 125–136.

Lee, L., Yang, K., Lee, C., & Wu, S. (2001). An evaluation of the effects of the implementation of UBSG on nurses' perceptions of professional governance [Chinese]. *Journal of Nursing Research* (China) 9(1): 5–13.

Lynn, J., Baily, M. A., Bottrell, M., Jennings, B., Levine, R. J. Davidoff, F., &James, B. (2007). The ethics of using quality improvement methods in health care. *Annals of Internal Medicine* 146: 666–673.

MacDonald, C. (2002). Nurse autonomy as relational. *Nursing Ethics* 9: 194–201.

Mallik, M., & Raffert, A. (2000). Diffusion of the concept of patient advocacy. *Journal of Nursing Scholarship* 32(4): 399–404.

Maxwell, J. C. (2007). *Failing Forward: Turning Mistakes Into Stepping Stones for Success.* Nashville: Thomas Nelson Publishers.

McClure, M. L., & Hinshaw, A. S. (Eds.) (2002). *Magnet Hospitals Revisited.* Washington, DC: American Nurses Publishing.

McDonagh, K., Rhodes, B., Sharkey, K., & Goodroe, J. (1989). Shared governance at Saint Joseph's hospital of Atlanta: A mature professional practice model. *Nursing Administration Quarterly* 13(4): 17–28.

Merton, R. (1960). The search for professional status. *American Journal of Nursing* 60: 662–664.

Metcalf, R., & Tate, R. (1995). Shared governance in the endoscopy department. *Gastroenterology Nursing* 18(3): 96–99.

Minnen, T., Berger, E., Ames, A., Dubree, M., Baker, W., & Spinella, J. (1993). Sustaining work redesign innovations through shared governance. *Journal of Nursing Administration* 23(7/8): 35–40.

Monaghan, H. M., & Swihart, D. (2010). *Clinical Nurse Leader: Transforming Practice, Transforming Care: A Model for the Clinician at the Point of Care.* Sarasota, FL: Visioning HealthCare, Inc.

Myhrberg, E. V. (2009). *A Practical Field Guide for ISO 9001:2008.* Milwaukee: ASQ Quality Press.

National Press Publications (Ed.). (2001). *The Manager's Role as Coach: Motivate, Mentor and Coach Your Most Valuable Asset—Your People—to Achieve Professional Excellence* (2nd ed.). Shawnee Mission, KS: National Press Publications, Inc.

National Quality Forum. (2004). *National Voluntary Consensus Standards for Nursing Home Care.* Washington DC: Author.

Needleman, J., Buerhaus, P., Matke, S., Stewart, M., & Zelevinsky, K. (2002). Nurse-staffing levels and the quality of care in hospitals. *New England Journal of Medicine* 346(22): 1715–1722.

Nightingale, F. (1992). *Notes on Nursing: What It Is, and What It Is Not.* Philadelphia: Lippincott Williams & Wilkins.

Nursing Executive Center Practice Brief. (2005). *Toward Staff-Driven Decision Making. Assessing, Building, and Sustaining a Shared Governance Model.* Washington, DC: The Advisory Board Company. (Entire IPNG included.)

O'May, F., & Buchan, J. (1999). Shared governance: A literature review. *International Journal of Nursing Studies* 36: 281–300.

Page, A. (Ed.) (2004). *Keeping Patients Safe: Transforming the Work Environment of Nurses.* Washington, DC: National Academy Press.

Perley, M. J., & Raab, A. (1994). Beyond shared governance: Restructuring care delivery for self-managing work teams. *Nursing Administration Quarterly* 19(1): 12–20.

Peterman, M. (2011). *Managing Change: Getting People to Want to Do What You Want Them To.* Presentation by Dr. Michael Peterman, Organizational Development Psychologist, at the Denver OCCC. Washington, DC: National Office of Clinical Consultation and Compliance.

Peters, T. J., & Waterman, Jr., R. H. (1982). *In Search of Excellence: Lessons From America's Best-Run Companies.* New York: Warner Books.

Peterson, M. E., & Allen, D. G. (1986a). Shared governance: A strategy for transforming organizations, Part 1. *Journal of Nursing Administration* 16(1): 9–12.

Peterson, M. E., & Allen, D. G. (1986b). Shared governance: A strategy for transforming organizations, Part 2. *Journal of Nursing Administration* 16(2): 11–16.

Pettitt, L. (2002). *Nursing Governance and Staff Nurses Self-Concept*. Master's thesis. Boiling Springs, NC: Gardner-Webb University.

Pittman, E. (2006). *Luther Christman: A Maverick Nurse—A Nursing Legend*. Bloomington, IN: Trafford Publishing.

Polit, D., & Beck, C. T. (2011). *Resource Manual for Nursing Research: Generating and Assessing Evidence for Nursing Practice*. Philadelphia: Lippincott Williams & Wilkins.

Porter-O'Grady, T. (1986). *Creative Nursing Administration: Managing Participation Into the Twenty First Century*. Rockville, MD: Aspen Publishers, Inc.

Porter-O'Grady, T. (1987). Shared governance and new organizational models. *Nursing Economic$* 5(6): 281–286.

Porter-O'Grady, T. (1989). Shared governance: Reality or sham? *American Journal of Nursing Administration* 89(3): 350–351.

Porter-O'Grady, T. (1990). *Reorganization of Nursing Practice: Creating the Corporate Venture*. Rockville, MD: Aspen Publications.

Porter-O'Grady, T. (1991). Shared governance for nursing part II: Putting the organization into action. *Association of periOperative Registered Nurses Journal* 53(3): 694–703.

Porter-O'Grady, T. (1992). *Implementing Shared Governance: Creating a Professional Organization*. St. Louis: Mosby-Year Books.

Porter-O'Grady, T. (2001). Is shared governance still relevant? *Journal of Nursing Administration* 31(10): 468–473.

Porter-O'Grady, T. (2002). "Nurses as partners." Hospitals and Health Networks/AHA, 76(12), 10, 12.

Porter-O'Grady, T. (2003a). A different age for leadership, Part 1: New context, new content. *Journal of Nursing Administration* 33(2): 105–110.

Porter-O'Grady, T. (2003b). A different age for leadership, Part 2: New rules, new roles. *Journal of Nursing Administration* 33(3): 173–178.

Porter-O'Grady, T. (2003c). Researching shared governance: A futility of focus. *Journal of Nursing Administration* 33(4): 251–252.

Porter-O'Grady, T. (2004). *Shared Governance Implementation Manual*. Atlanta: Tim Porter-O'Grady Associates, Inc.

Porter-O'Grady, T. (2007a). Part V. 4. A capital transformation. In S. M. Weinstein & A. T. Brooks (Eds.), *Nursing Without Borders: Values, Wisdom, Success Markers*, pp 201–207. Indianapolis: Sigma Theta Tau International.

Porter-O'Grady, T. (2007b). Innovation, architecture and quantum reality: Synthesis in a new age for healthcare. *Health Environments Research and Design Journal* 1(1): 17–19.

Porter-O'Grady, T. (2007c). Push parameters forward using evidence-based approaches. *Nursing Management* 38(6): 58, 60–61

Porter-O'Grady, T. (2007d). The CNO as entrepreneur: Innovation leadership for a new age. *Nursing Administration Quarterly* 5(1): 44–47

Porter-O'Grady, T. (March 2008). Creating an innovative nursing organization, *AONE Voice of Nursing Leadership* (March 2008). (PDF available at *www.tpogassociates.com/reference/2008/innovativenursing.pdf*.) Accessed online May 14, 2011.

Porter-O'Grady, T. (2009a). Creating a context for excellence: Comparing chief nurse executive leadership practices in Magnet and non-Magnet hospitals. *Nursing Administration Quarterly* 33(3): 198–204.

Porter-O'Grady, T. (2009b). Innovation, leadership and organizational transformation. *Nursing Administration Quarterly* referenced and accessed online May 14, 2011 at *www.tpogassociates.com/publications.htm*.

Porter-O'Grady, T. (2009c). *Interdisciplinary Shared Governance: Structuring for 21st Century Practice*. Sudbury, MA: Jones & Bartlett Publishers.

Porter-O'Grady, T. (2009d). Leadership for excellence issue. *Nursing Administration Quarterly* referenced and accessed online May 14, 2011 at *www.tpogassociates.com/publications.htm*.

Porter-O'Grady, T. (July 2010a). Challenging regulation realities in a new age for practice. *Journal of Nursing Regulation*, 1(2), 4–7.

Porter-O'Grady, T. (2010b). Nurses as knowledge workers. In L. Caputi (Ed.), *Teaching Nursing: The Art and Science*, vol. 2, pp. 356–380. Glen Ellyn, IL: College of Dupage Press.

Porter-O'Grady, T. (2010c). *Quantum Leadership: Advancing Innovation, Transforming Healthcare* (3rd ed.). Sudbury, MA: Jones & Bartlett Publishers.

Porter-O'Grady, T., & Basinger, S. (2010). Chapter 10. A transformational moment, In N. R. Gantz (Ed.), *101 Global Leadership Lessons for Nurses: Shared Legacies From Leaders and Their Mentors*, pp. 50–54. Indianapolis, IN: Sigma Theta Tau International.

Porter-O'Grady, T., Clark, J. S., & Wiggins, M. S. (2010). The case for clinical nurse leaders: Guiding practice into the 21st century. *AONE Journal* 8(1): 37–41.

Porter-O'Grady, T., & Finnigan, S. (1984). *Shared Governance for Nursing: A Creative Approach to Professional Accountability*. Rockville, MD: Aspen Systems Corp.

Porter-O'Grady, T., Hawkins, M. A., & Parker, M. L. (Eds.). (1997). *Whole-Systems Shared Governance: Architecture for Integration*. Gaithersburg, MD: Aspen Publishers.

Porter-O'Grady, T., & Hitchings, K. S. (2005). *Shared Governance: How to Create and Sustain a Culture of Nurse Empowerment* (Audioconference). Marblehead, MA: HCPro, Inc.

Porter-O'Grady, T., & Malloch, K. (2009). *Innovation Leadership*. Sudbury, MA: Jones & Bartlett Publishers.

Porter-O'Grady, T., & Malloch, K. (2003). *Quantum Leadership: A Textbook of New Leadership*. Sudbury, MA: Jones & Bartlett Publishers.

Porter-O'Grady, T., & Malloch, K. (2009). *The Quantum Leader: Applications for the New World of Work.* Sudbury, MA: Jones & Bartlett Publishers.

Porter-O'Grady, T., & Malloch, K. (2010a). Innovation: Driving the Green Culture in Healthcare. *Nursing Administration Quarterly.*

Porter-O'Grady, T., & Malloch, K. (2010b). *The Leadership of Innovation: Transforming Healthcare.* Sudbury, MA: Jones & Bartlett Publishers.

Porter-O'Grady, T., & Malloch, K. (2010c). *Principles of Evidence-Based Practice* (2nd ed.). Sudbury, MA: Jones & Bartlett Publishers.

Porter-O'Grady, T., & McNeil, A. (2007). Engaging transformation: Constructing a new model for nursing education and practice. *Nurse Leader* 5(30): 30–34.

Porter-O'Grady, T., & Wilson, C. (1995). *The Leadership Revolution in Health Care: Altering Systems Changing Behavior.* Rockville, MD: Aspen Publishers.

Porter-O'Grady, T., & Wilson, C. (1998, 2008). *The Healthcare TEAMbook.* St. Louis: Mosby Books (1998), TPOG Inc. (2008).

Prince, S. B. (1997). Shared governance: Sharing power and opportunity. *Journal of Nursing Administration* 27(3), 28–35.

Richards, K. C., Ragland, P., Zehler, J., Dotson, K., Berube, M., Tygart, M. W., Gibson, R. A. (1999). Implementing a councilor model: Process and outcomes. *Journal of Nursing Administration* 29(7/8): 19–27.

Rocchiccioli, J., & Tilbury, M. S. (1998). *Clinical Leadership in Nursing.* Philadelphia: W. B. Saunders/Elsevier Publishing.

Sabiston, J. A., & Lashinger, H. K. S. (1995). Staff nurse work empowerment and perceived autonomy. *Journal of Nursing Administration* 25(9): 42–50.

Sackett, D. L., Straus, S. E., Richardson, W. S., Rosenberg, W., & Haynes, R. B. (2000). *Evidence-Based Medicine: How to Practice and Teach EBM* (2nd ed.). Edinburgh: Churchill Livingstone.

Schoemer, K. G. (2009). *Change Is Your Competitive Advantage: Strategies for Adapting, Transforming, and Succeeding in the New Business Reality.* Avon, MA: Adams Media.

Scott, J., & Marshall, G. (Eds). (2005). *A Dictionary of Sociology.* New York: Oxford University Press.

Senge, P., Kleiner, A., Roberts, C., Ross, R. B., & Smith, B. J. (1994). *The Fifth Discipline Fieldbook: Strategies and Tools for Building a Learning Organization.* New York: Doubleday.

Singh, R. (2010). *Shared Governance as a Source of Nurse Empowerment.* Doctoral capstone. Fort Lauderdale, FL: Florida Atlantic University.

Song, R., Daly, B. J., Rudy, E. B., Douglas, S., & Dyer, M. A. (1997). Nurses' job satisfaction, absenteeism, and turnover after implementing a special care unit practice model. *Research in Nursing and Health* 20: 443–452.

Staff. (1996). Interview of Robert Hess and Tim Porter-O'Grady addressing 13 questions concerning the progress and future of shared governance. *Journal of Shared Governance* 2(4): 11–15.

Stumpf, L. R. (2001). A comparison of governance types and patient satisfaction outcomes. *Journal of Nursing Administration* 31(4): 196–202.

Swihart, D. (2006). *Shared Governance. A Practical Approach to Reshaping Professional Nursing Practice.* Marblehead, MA: HCPro, Inc. (Entire IPNG and IPG included.)

Swihart, D. (2011). *Shared Governance. A Practical Approach to Transform Professional Nursing Practice.* Danvers, MA: HCPro. (Entire IPNG and IPG included.)

The Advisory Board Company. (2005). Best practice solutions to health care's most pressing challenges. Washington, DC. Accessed May 14, 2011 online at accessible online at *www.advisoryboardcompany.com*.

The Greenleaf Center for Servant Leadership. Retrieved from *www.greenleaf.org*.

Upenieks, V. V. (2003). What constitutes effective leadership? Perceptions of Magnet and nonMagnet nurse leaders. *The Journal of Nursing Administration* 33: 456–467.

Urden, L. D., & Monarch, K. (2002). The ANCC Magnet Recognition Program: Converting research findings into action. In M. L. McClure & A. S. Hinshaw (Eds.), *Magnet Hospitals Revisited: Attraction and Retention of Professional Nurses* (pp. 103–116). Washington, DC: American Nurse Association.

U.S. Department of Health and Human Services. (n.d.). *Code of Federal Regulations Title 45 Public Welfare Part 46: Protection of Human Subjects, Title 21 Food and Drugs Part 50: Protection of Human Subjects.* Washington, DC: Author.

Walter, M. R., Aucoin, J., Brown, R., Thompson, J., & Sullivan, D. T. (Jan 2014). A multimodal approach to EBP. *Nursing Management* 45(1), 14–17.

Weinberg, D. B. (2003). *Code Green: Money-Driven Hospitals and the Dismantling of Nursing.* Ithaca, NY: Cornell University Press.

Weston, M. (2006). *Antecedents to Control Over Nursing Practice.* Doctoral dissertation. Tucson, AZ: College of Nursing, University of Arizona.

Wright, D. (2002). R + A + A: The secret formula for making communication and delegation easier. Video 4 in the *Moments of Excellence* video series. Minneapolis: Creative Health Care Management.

Wright, D. (2005). *The Ultimate Guide to Competency Assessment* (3rd ed.). Minneapolis: Creative Health Care Management.